Praise for *AIDS Orphans Rising*

Every 15 seconds.... Every 15 seconds a new Child-Headed Household comes into being in the poorest parts of the world. More than 13 million children struggle for survival without both parents due to AIDS. *AIDS Orphans Rising* is a rigorously researched, compelling, carefully chronicled call to action and labor of love of Sister Mary Elizabeth Lloyd, MPF. In the time it took to write these sentences, another Child-Headed Household was born. That's the point. Sister Mary Beth stirs the embers on every person's possibility to make some difference in addressing this crisis. The inclusion of the orphans' personal stories and photos bring the text to life. *Every 15 seconds.* In the time it took to read this blub another child is orphaned and becomes the head of her or his band of siblings in search of daily bread and hope.

> Avis Clendenen, D.Min., Ph.D. Professor Emerita
> Saint Xavier University/Chicago

Though the western world hardly talks any more about people with AIDS, tens of millions of AIDS orphans are left to fend for themselves in the Third World. Filippini Sister Mary Elizabeth Lloyd shares firsthand experience how her religious community cares for them and invites the rest of the world to join in. Her scientific and health backgrounds expose the enormity of the problem. Her compassionate conscience shames the world to a human problem it cannot ignore.

> Fr. Alexander M. Santora, Catholic pastor
> and "Faith Matters" columnist for *The Jersey Journal*

I personally know Sister Mary Elizabeth and totally endorse her and her book. She is coming from her heart and sincerely wants to make a difference in the world. This book is a treasure and a guide.

> Joe Vitale, author of *The Key*, costar in *The Secret*

Sr. Mary Elizabeth has gifted us with a marvelous book! Her scientific study on the crisis of AIDS in children of underdeveloped countries is written in a compassionate, caring manner that deeply touches and moves the heart of the reader. It is a book that will affect you profoundly. I am proud and honored to commend this outstanding work.

> Sister Mary De Bacco, M.P.F., Superior General emerita

Here is a realistic, meticulously-researched look at the problems faced by the millions of AIDS orphans in Africa, and the people who are attempting to care for them. But even more, this is a story of the transcendence of the human spirit, as we learn about children facing their challenges with incredible resilience, determination, and yes—even joy. We in the west must not give up on them, because they are certainly not giving up on themselves.

Jillian C. Wheeler, CEO, author, philanthropist

This book is an inspiring gem of human caring for human. Particularly, the last chapter is beautiful and inspiring. It is very clearly written, and for the ordinary reader, and yet it is a fully documented scholarly work.

Bob Rich, PhD, author *Cancer: A Personal Challenge*

AIDS Orphans Rising will grip your heart. The needs will linger in your consciousness long after you have read the final word and closed the covers of the book. Sister Mary Elizabeth Lloyd has presented the case for these children. Now it is up to us, the readers, to decide which suggested action steps we can take to help them succeed.

Richard Blake, *Reader Views*

Parents want to teach their children to be compassionate toward others. School and youth groups are always looking for worthy projects. Adults can get the book, share with the children whatever information they believe is appropriate for their age, and then work together to come up with ways to assist. This is not a "fun" or pleasant book to read, but it contains information about our world, however heart-wrenching it may be, which we and our children need to know in order to love our neighbors as ourselves.

Virginia S Grenier, *Stories For Children*

AIDS Orphans Rising:

What You Should Know and What You Can Do to Help Them Succeed, 2nd Edition

Sister Mary Elizabeth Lloyd, MPF, EdD

Foreword by Connie Mariano, MD, FACP

Loving Healing Press
Ann Arbor, MI

AIDS Orphans Rising: What You Should Know and What You Can Do to Help Them Succeed, 2nd Edition

ISBN 978-1-61599-399-4 eBook
ISBN 978-1-61599-400-7 hardcover
ISBN 978-1-61599-401-4 paperback

Library of Congress Cataloging-in-Publication Data

Names: Lloyd, Mary Elizabeth, author.
Title: AIDS orphans rising : what you should know and what you can do to help
    them succeed, 2nd edition / by Sister Mary Elizabeth Lloyd ; foreword by
    Connie Mariano.
Description: 2nd edition. | Ann Arbor : Loving Healing Press, 2018. |
    Includes bibliographical references and index.
Identifiers: LCCN 2018029877 (print) | LCCN 2018031488 (ebook) | ISBN
    9781615993994 (Kindle, ePub, pdf) | ISBN 9781615994007 (case-laminate
    hardcover : alk. paper) | ISBN 9781615994014 (trade pbk. : alk. paper)
Subjects: LCSH: AIDS (Disease)--Social aspects. | Children of AIDS patients.
    | Orphans. | Youth-headed households.
Classification: LCC RA643.8 (ebook) | LCC RA643.8 .L66 2018 (print) | DDC
    362.1969792--dc23

Published by:
Loving Healing Press
5145 Pontiac Trail
Ann Arbor, MI 48105

www.LHPress.com
info@LHPress.com
Tollfree 888-761-6268 (USA, CAN, PR)
Fax 734-663-6861

Distributed by Ingram Book Group (USA/CAN/AU), Bertram's Books
(UK/EU).

Contents

Pictures in this Book

Foreword

This slender sheet of glass is all that separates me from these children. I remember the experience like it was yesterday. It was an epiphany I encountered while riding in the decoy limousine as White House physician for President Bill Clinton during a motorcade through the densely crowded, sweltering Tondo district of Manila. The vehicle was swarmed by hundreds of poor children, each of them in need. This window, made from darkly tinted, durable, bulletproof glass, failed to block the horrific impact of third world hunger and poverty. I tried to wave back in a friendly way, but there was nothing for me to do. There was no way to open the window. And if I could, what good would it do anyway? Fast forward to today, reading *AIDS Orphans Rising* can open many windows.

I was first introduced to Sister Mary Elizabeth Lloyd, MPF (hereafter Sister Mary Beth) through a medical school classmate, and learned about the global ministry of her teaching order, the Religious Teachers Filippini. Its foundress, Saint Lucy Filippini, was orphaned in childhood in Italy over three centuries ago. Poverty and illiteracy were rampant across Italy at that time. Lucy Filippini was the forerunner of today's women's empowerment movement. She collaborated with Cardinal Mark Anthony Barbarigo, and together they opened 52 schools. These schools promoted the dignity of womanhood and helped influence a healthy family life. Lucy organized classes and conferences that guided women in prayer, meditation and good works. Her focus for the social apostolate was to encourage her teachers to minister to the needs of the poor and the sick. Today, the Religious Teachers Filippini support women and children on five continents, and Sister Mary Beth serves as their International Missions Director. How humbling it is to be involved in this beautiful ministry.

I personally know the face of poverty. It is the face of my father who was born in the Philippines close to 94 years ago, into a family of seven children. While his father was away on the island of Corregidor, sewing uniforms for American soldiers, my father's mother delivered her eighth newborn in the family's bamboo hut, attended by the village midwife. The baby boy entered the world stillborn. As soon as he was delivered, my paternal grandmother began to hemorrhage from a ruptured placenta; her blood dripping through the slats of the bamboo floor. Her seven children, including my father who was 11 years old at that time, witnessed their mother's last breath. My grandfather returned to their village three days later to find his wife lying in a casket, her deceased infant in her arms, surrounded by her weeping children.

As the family carried her casket to the church for the funeral Mass, the townspeople took pity upon my father and his siblings, saying, "This family was poor to begin with and now without their mother, they will be even more poor." The loss of one's mother is devastating to family and community. Now consider the loss of both parents, as has happened to the thousands of orphans depicted in this book; the scope of this catastrophe is beyond comprehension.

A decade ago, Sister Mary Beth published the first edition of *AIDS Orphans Rising* over concerns for the invisible (and exploding) crisis of child-headed households in Africa. It was originally intended to serve as a resource guidebook for concerned teachers, researchers, nonprofit organizations, and policymakers. A strange thing happened; other people began reading the book, too! Sister Mary Beth has many beautiful stories of generous strangers, young and old, who have approached her to offer help. As a result, the perspective of this second edition has been reframed to inform concerned citizens everywhere. It is less didactic and far more accessible than the original work. There is more narrative and more storytelling to go along with the many updated resources and weblinks.

Has anything changed regarding the crisis in Africa over the past decade? Sadly, the rate of new child-headed households has not slowed appreciably, and the AIDS epidemic continues in Africa. The youngsters portrayed in the first edition are now young adults, and many of them have acquired HIV. It is a cycle that will continue until sufficient resources are mobilized and effectively managed.

Two key takeaway lessons from this informative book are awareness of the global proliferation of child-headed households, and the continuing need to address the spread of HIV. It is such a colossal undertaking, but as both Mother Teresa and Sister Mary Beth espouse: Nobody can do it all, but everybody can do one thing, one small thing.

During my career, I've been blessed to be in the company of amazing thinkers and leaders—heads of state, academic geniuses, medical innovators, successful entrepreneurs, and more. These phenomenal people champion successful endeavors by uniting populations and organizations to accomplish great things. I include Sister Mary Beth among these remarkable people, however, her paradigm for success begins within the individual—and so does peace.

Connie Mariano, MD, FACP
Rear Admiral, US Navy, Retired
Former Director, White House Medical Unit
Former White House Physician to Presidents
George H.W. Bush and Bill Clinton

How This Book Began

I had been struggling with the world's continued nonchalance toward children orphaned by AIDS, so it was a true gift when I was asked to write a second edition of *AIDS Orphans Rising*. When I started this work in 1994, a Child-Headed Household was formed every 14 seconds. Things have gotten better—today it is every 15 seconds! That means children, usually very young and by the thousands, are being left alone to fend for themselves. How can this be? How can it be that in a world with robots, self-driving cars, and wonderful doctors and scientists, we still do not have a cure for AIDS? And, sadly, people in remote parts of the world have no access to education about the disease, not to mention medicine. For many in these countries, AIDS is still the "skinny disease" that takes the father first, then the newest baby, then the mother. The remaining siblings are left to care for themselves. There are millions of orphans out there. My hope is that this book will help these children in need. Let me share with you how this work began decades ago.

In 1995, retrieving my suitcase from the hall, after having just arrived from a 14-hour flight and three-hour van ride to Adigrat, Ethiopia from the USA, I heard a faint knock at the door. Upon opening it, I found two little boys. One said, "My name is Moses. And the other, in a very frail manner said, "I'm Abraham." Biblical names, was my first thought!

Moses, who looked about nine years old, meekly said, "We are students in your school. Could you help us? Our older sister left us this morning after our brother, who was just released from prison, took all of our food and money!"

This was quite a story for me to digest after a long journey. I called Sister Lette, who said she would give them some food, and then later we could visit with them at their home. Sr. Lette told me that they had lost their parents to HIV/AIDS. She was quick to add, "There are about 600 children like this in town and 70,000 in the Diocese of Adigrat."

Later that afternoon, we walked over to see how the boys were doing. Sister explained that, until today, the family of Moses and Abraham were "*on the rise.*" The two boys were doing well in our elementary school. Abraham, (see Pic. I-1), was being treated by the doctor for his tuberculosis of the bone, but able to go to school each day. His older sister was in our program where she was working for her elementary school diploma and also receiving training in operating an industrial knitting machine. She was on her way to having her own business. Like so many of the orphans, they were working hard to have a great life. We can help them, and all others like them, to acquire the skills that would enable them to care for their siblings in a sustainable way.

We, the Religious Teachers Filippini, have been helping the women and children of the Tigray Region of Ethiopia and Eritrea to succeed in life through our elementary schools and women promotion centers for almost 50 years. We have seen the effects of wars and famines, but never, never, have we experienced anything like this!

This small family was my introduction to the little-known phenomenon of Child-Headed Households (hereafter referred to as CHH), one of which is formed every 15 seconds.

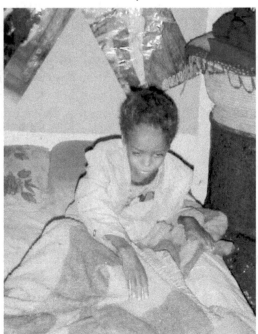

Pic. I-1: Abraham, alone again with tuberculosis of the bone.

The growing phenomenon of these children scraping for survival shows the determination of the remnants of families to stay together. My experience with the children in India and Brazil was very different, with many children orphaned, but not living with siblings.

Why do the African orphan siblings fight to survive together? Often alienated by the stigma of parents who have died of AIDS, the orphan families of Ethiopia carry on working the farm and attending school. These children are Africa's chance to break the cycle of poverty that has held a grip on the continent for centuries. With help from people who believe in them, and a good education, these courageous and determined children will show us all what good can be accomplished. They possess strength, and qualities of leadership that need to be nurtured and encouraged. My hope is that this book will enable you to understand the plight of these children, and encourage you to help them to succeed.

Introduction

AIDS Orphans Rising will introduce you to real children, orphaned by AIDS, who are struggling to keep their family together. Most policy guidelines for children portray them as victims who are dependent and powerless. Little attention has been given to the positive aspects of these children's behavior, and how they have been able to take control of their lives.

In this book, you will see brothers and sisters from one to eighteen years of age fighting all the odds to stay together. **It is not a sad story**. For them, this is life. They see people struggling all around them, but they see those who get up and go survive. It is a tremendous story of courage, of children willing to forego education and their childhood itself, for the sake of love for their family. This is the story of children, who with a little help and love, will grow up to be fine citizens of the 21st century.

Statistics from around the world have been included so that you may see the vastness of this problem. Hopefully, it might touch your heart, and motivate you to use your talents to help these children. We, who have had a wonderful childhood, brought up by loving and protective parents, have the knowledge and wherewithal to reach out to these children. Those of you reading who perhaps did not have the best parents in the world, at least had healthcare and school, something these children may never receive without your help.

My hope is that reading this work will be beneficial to you, as many of us know little of the plight or successes of these children. Yes, television and concerts are great at telling you there is an AIDS crisis and there are orphans. You see them poor and hungry and helpless at a quick glance, but this book will allow you to see more closely, not just what these children are up against, but how they can succeed and how you can make a difference in their lives.

Many people believe HIV infection levels are exaggerated. According to estimates by the World Health Organization (WHO) and UNAIDS, there were approximately 36.7 million people living with HIV at the end of 2016, with 1.8 million people becoming newly infected in 2016 globally. The WHO African Region is the most affected, with 25.6 million people living with HIV in 2016. The African region also accounts for almost two thirds of the global total of new HIV infections.

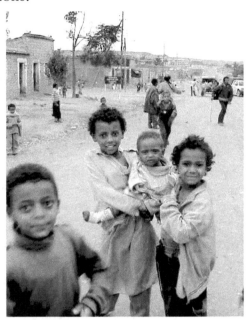

Pic. I-2: Meet Tsefy, Desta, Leo and Anna. They have been living on their own since their mother died, giving birth to Anna.

There are 18.8 million women and girls living with HIV, with more than 2.1 million of them under 15 years of age. Consequently, thousands of young children are newly infected with the virus each day.

Can you visualize how quickly the virus can spread? The geometric progression continues at a greater speed among populations affected by AIDS. As the number of infected adults rises, so too does the number of AIDS orphans increase. Today, a new Child-Headed Household is formed every 15 seconds.

Many of the infected men and women have little access to life-extending drugs. Soon, most of the mothers and fathers will die, leaving behind not only their babies, but also those babies' siblings, all of them now orphans.

In November, 2016, UNICEF updated its *Current Status and Progress Report*. This *Report* provides the broadest and most comprehensive statistics yet on the historical, current, and projected number of children orphaned by HIV/AIDS.

The following chart shows only several countries, but they account for millions of orphans. These are the documented orphans; there are millions more throughout the world still unaccounted for.

Country	Children Orphaned by AIDS
South Africa	2,300,000
Tanzania	1,300,000
Kenya	1,000,000
Uganda	650,000
Mozambique	610,000
Zimbabwe	570,000
Malawi	530,000
Ethiopia	450,000
Zambia	380,000
Congo	290,000
World Total	**8,080,000**

A great many diverse areas need attention and help within the tragedy of AIDS orphans. This book is not about *street kids* living alone, or about orphans with AIDS. **It's about healthy brothers and sisters who have lost their parents from AIDS and are striving to keep together what remains of their family.**

How these children are helped will directly influence the kind of adults they become, the country they inherit, and the world. These are the next generation of voters, taxpayers, leaders, and parents. If we fail to provide for the spiritual, moral, emotional, psychological and physical needs of these children, not only will we have failed them personally, but one can imagine the chaos that will descend upon us and future generations, affecting all the countries of the world for many years to come. What is to stop these lost children from becoming jihadists? Only love!

Families are the bedrock from which everything else flows, and if you have a family or people who love you, you can carry on and even do much good in this world. Historians one hundred years from now will regard the HIV/AIDS epidemic as a fundamental determinant for most of the history of the 21st century. As you learn of these children, please pray for them, think how you might use your talents to help them, and act on it.

1 What is a Child-Headed Household?

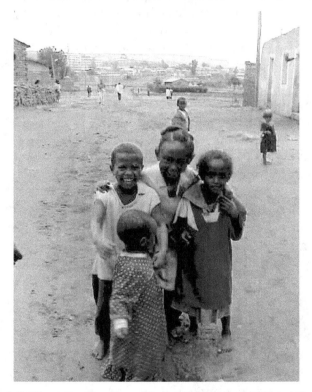

Pic. 1-1: Meet the Family – Abeba, Dawit, Emebet and Feker.
This is a Child-Headed Household.

Every day, thousands of Child-Headed Households are formed. You may wonder what, exactly, is a Child-Headed Household or CHH? It is a family of siblings who have survived the death of their parents and now live with the eldest sibling as head of the household. The eldest sibling in a Child-Headed Household is under the age of eighteen. A CHH is comprised of brothers and sisters, like Abeba, Dawit, Emebet and Feker, who are struggling to stay alive and remain together as a family (see Pic. 1-1). Since *both* parents of these four siblings have died, they might be referred to as "double orphans." This is not a new phenomenon to history. In previous eras, most Child-Headed Households came about because the parents died as a result of war. Today there are still CHH being formed by the tragedy of war, but now half of all CHH are formed because the parents have died from HIV/AIDS. You can find a brief overview of HIV/AIDS in Appendix A.

The orphans of war cry often, and frequently tell their stories over and over to anyone who will listen, especially when they get back to school. They tell their classmates what happened to their parents. Perhaps a bomb hit the house, or their father was killed by a gunshot. These orphans have a particular way of expressing their sorrow, and the other children in their class respect them because they have survived the tragedy of war.

However, unlike war orphans, the orphaned children of the Bililla family cry silently behind closed doors. They have no one to tell their story to, because there are so many children in the same situation. No one wants to hear the details of a far too familiar story. The neighbors all know that the children's parents died from what they call "the skinny disease." All have watched the children struggle through their parents' sickness and horrible agonizing death. When Emebet, David and Feker get to school, they will just go inside, put their heads on their desks, and cry. The other children rarely sympathize because most of them have been through the same tragedy. It's more like they will tell them, "Get over it. We're all in the same boat." The Bililla children cannot grieve like the children orphaned by war, but must get on with life and make a living or die. It is almost impossible to believe that the eldest sibling in this family is only ten years old.

Emebet, the oldest daughter, is responsible for her three siblings. Their parents must have been a loving couple before passing away from AIDS. Listen to their children's names and what they mean: Abeba, the smallest child in the picture, means flower; Dawit, the only son, means beloved; next is Emebet, which means respected first lady; and last is Feker, which means love. But how did their parents get the AIDS virus? It is thought that something went wrong on the farm, perhaps crop failure from the drought, so their father took the truck and went to work in the capital, Addis Abbaba. While there, he fooled around with another woman, even though he loved his wife, and contracted the AIDS virus. Weeks later he returned to his family and, after awhile, he and his wife conceived a baby. Unbeknownst to him, he passed the virus on to both of them. All were dead within five years, leaving behind the Child-Headed Household pictured below.

Mr. Bililla and his wife did not make any alternative living arrangements for their children. Both were so sick, and living in such terrible conditions, that they didn't have the strength or wherewithal to plan for the future of their family. They believed that, should they die, the grandparents or extended family members would provide for the children. Now left alone, the Bililla children must provide for themselves. Many of the children in these circumstances resort to begging for money for food and clothing. Some girls resort to prostitution to raise money. Fetching water, cooking and cleaning are all shared tasks among the children. They face daily threats to their survival.

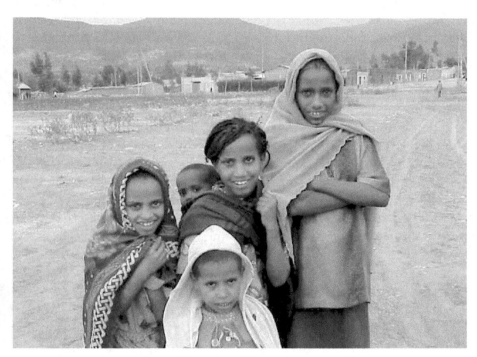

**Pic. 1-2: Meet Fikre, the oldest girl responsible for:
Rada, Zahra, Neguse, & Hanna.**

Fikre (see Pic. 1-2) takes her role as mother and breadwinner through a natural sequence of events. When talking about her situation, she is rather matter of fact. The tears come, but she keeps telling you what she has in mind for the day and how she will provide for her brothers and sisters. There is no self-pity, just goodness and the desire to make certain that her siblings have a good upbringing.

Traditional coping mechanisms are being threatened as communities are overwhelmed with the enormous scale of this problem. These are children who plead for medicines for their mothers and fathers and cannot get them. Tragically, they must watch their parents die long and agonizing deaths. This leaves the orphaned children without the critical guidance, protection and support required for a successful and healthy life.

The children witness the family struggling and disintegrating before their eyes. They see the household food source and any meager income disappear. Many are forced to leave school. Some feel forlorn, terrified and abandoned when death claims its victims. But, there are also encouraging stories. Some orphans, because of guidance from their parents before their death, are able to cope, and show a resilience to get back into life and make it better for all.

Young Joseph's father taught him how to slaughter a cow and divide it into steaks and ribs, and even how to tan leather for shoes. When his mom and dad passed away, Joseph continued what his dad had taught him and provided food not only for his siblings, but also for the village. Because there is no refrigeration, the CHHs who received the meat would all cook it the same night. The village smelled like barbecue heaven! So you can see that, despite the poor odds, there are success stories.

Even the smallest assistance can make a great impact. For example, young Grace was good at sewing and wanted to make covers for people's cell phones. She had noticed how dirty the phones would get from the dusty streets. Then, someone gave her money for cloth. At first she sold five covers, then ten, and then had orders for so many covers, she had to hire other girls to help her. Now Grace is able to provide for her siblings, and the friends she hires are also sustaining their younger brothers and sisters.

CHH are usually comprised of three to eight children per household. The head of most CHH is usually from 10 to 14 years old. And, girls lead three quarters of all CHH. Pic. 1-2 shows the Alazar family. This is a CHH led by an eleven-year-old girl, Fikre. She is trying to raise her two younger sisters, Hanna and Zahra, and her two younger brothers, Rada and Neguse, to grow up and receive an education. Fikre and her siblings have the emotional needs common to children everywhere.

Unfortunately, they will never receive much needed emotional counseling.

The millions of children in CHH need our support, so they can remain in charge of their lives without fear of being split up or sent away. They face so many challenges. Because many of them are less than five years old, the orphan children encounter frequent illnesses and experience high mortality rates. They are exposed to a poor environment, malnutrition, and lack of medical attention, which further compromises their quality of life.

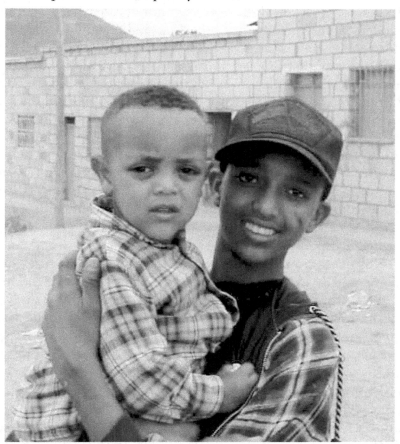

Pic. 1-3: Mekonnen, 14-years-old, responsible his 5-year-old brother.

Meet another CHH: the Senai Family. Mekonnen is holding his five-year-old brother Girma, in Pic. 1-3. Fourteen-year-old Mekonnen is treated as a young adult and expected to behave as a mature grownup. Adolescents from 11 to 15 years of age are in a crucial stage of their social development process and they need parental guidance. As much as he tries to work and provide some leadership for his brother, Mekonnen is still a child, and not ready for parenthood. He needs guidance, time, and a chance to be a teenager and experience this important stage of human development. The death of his father deprived Mekonnen of a male authority, a status symbol in many communities. But the subsequent death of his mother further deprived him of crucial emotional and mental security as well. This is the situation of hundreds of thousands of teenagers leading a CHH.

With help, however, these orphan children can achieve success. As mentioned in the introduction, the first CHH family I met was in trouble because their fifteen-year-old brother came home from prison, took all the money from the house, and ran away. But not all boys respond that way. Tomaso was fourteen years old and very good at math. One of the Sisters at school invited him to work on her computer. She taught him how to use the program Microsoft Excel. Tomaso would go to the stores in town and tell the owners that he would do their books and bring them a spreadsheet. He acquired so many clients that he was able to get his own computer and printer. He's now on his way to being a successful accountant!

While Tomaso's story is encouraging, most CHH are unfortunately not so lucky. Most are deprived of love, security, and a sense of belonging, acceptance and care. They have no one to turn to, and live in very difficult circumstances, without the basic necessities of life. They are usually exploited or taken advantage of; hence the loss of trust in the society that is supposed to protect them. Relatives or neighbors take most of the property left behind by their parents. Children in such conditions are deprived of their childhood and the opportunity to go to school. Economic hardships lead them to search for means of subsistence. This search often increases their vulnerability to HIV infection, substance abuse, child labor, sex work and delinquency.

Initially, the international community virtually ignored the issue of AIDS orphans, putting its efforts into AIDS prevention. There was a time when we believed that we could stop the epidemic. And today in the US you rarely hear of HIV/AIDS any more. But it still strongly ravages areas that have no access to the antiviral medicines. And not all of the orphans are CHH; many are out on their own. Most heart wrenching, upon arriving at the international airport in Mumbai at 2 AM it was necessary to get to the domestic airport for our trip to the state of

Andhra Pradesh. We got into the rickshaw and headed for the domestic airport. At the first red light, we were swarmed by hundreds of children, out on the streets at 2:00 a.m. They were hungry, and begging for food or money. We gave them the few sandwiches we had and some rupees.

The driver got out of the rickshaw with a stick and kept beating the children away until the traffic light changed. He said he brings the stick because this happens every time he stops at a light! Their faces are etched in my heart. How could we allow this to continue? Although the orphans I encountered in India were not CHH, they were still orphans trying to survive, exactly like the AIDS orphans in Ethiopia.

Even though these stories are often bleak, the Child-Headed Households of Ethiopia are an emerging positive outcome for affected communities. The term itself, Child-Headed Household, emphasizes the resilience and power of children heading families while living as orphans in challenging circumstances.

We cannot view these children as helpless! That would send a message to them that their own efforts to cope are not seen as legitimate, and would undermine their ability to succeed in overcoming the obstacles in their daily lives.

During my time in Ethiopia, I witnessed the daily lives of these orphaned children. I watched as they gathered their food, went to school, worked and played. And, despite all of the odds, so many do survive and thrive. Those who survive do so with the help of someone just like you. The following chapters will further explain how the children in a CHH live and, more important, how you can use your talents to help them succeed.

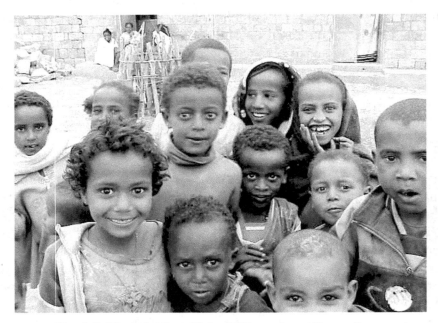

Pic. 1-4: Mimi, Jember, Fisha, Biftu and countless others.

2   Where Do They Live?

Finding a place to call home is a true challenge for the millions of Child-Headed Households. Eleven-year-old Beca and two-year-old Daniel sleep under a tarp in an alleyway and call it their home (see Pic. 2-1). Many, many CHH live in homes that are merely plastic tarps similar to those used to cover our boats in the winter.

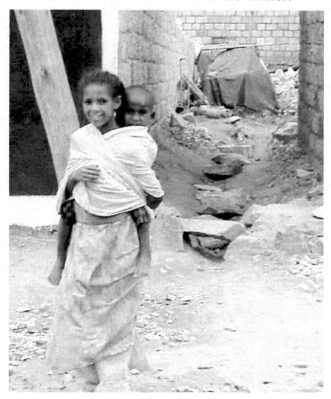

Pic. 2-1: For Beca and her younger brother Daniel, home is sleeping beneath a tarp.

The Dese family, eleven-year-old Zewdu, ten-year-old Ayara, and seven-year-old Fassil, have been sleeping in a cave since their parents died last year and they were forced off of the family farm. They huddle together for warmth. And another CHH, thirteen-year-old Ezera and his younger sisters, nine-year-old Candace, and seven-year-old Layla, sleep on the bare floor of a shop in town. They don't have a bed, mattress or blankets. Many others live in one-room homes where food is scarce. They often sleep on a flour sack, resting on the cement floor. For most of the orphans, there is no running water, no electricity, no bathrooms and no showers.

And despite these conditions, it is impressive to see how these children can make a one-room four-wall cement box home! They tape pictures on the walls and are sure to sweep it out each morning before going out to school or work. They stack any little items they may own neatly in boxes along the wall, and the last one out locks the door.

Type the phrase "children living in sewers" into Google search. You'll get more than 2 million hits! That's an increase of 400,000 since 2010. Watch the videos on YouTube that show you their living conditions. These children are not all orphans of AIDS (although many are), but *all* are homeless children in need of help. Tens of thousands of children live this way in Bucharest, Colombia, Mexico City, Bogata, and many large cities throughout the world.

When Jember's mother died at home, he and his two older brothers moved to live with their grandmother. Usually in such a situation they would move in with an aunt or uncle's family, but they had died from the virus, too.

Being raised by your grandparents is now known as "skip-generation parenting." The latest US Census data shows that in the United States there are approximately 2.7 million grandparents (up 7% since 2009) raising millions of children. Grandparent-headed orphan households are becoming increasingly common as a result of AIDS. For example, in Zimbabwe, 185,000 children are cared for by grandparents; and even in New York, 100,000 maternal orphans live with a grandmother.

Often, a grandparent cares for grandchildren from three or four families. The responsibility for orphan care is shifting increasingly to the grandmothers. The family networks are sagging under the weight of this epidemic. Many move in with grandparents whose desperate poverty only becomes worse with more mouths to feed.

The grandmother pictured at right (Pic. 2-2) had ten children. They grew up and got married. All of her children and their spouses have died from HIV/AIDS and Grandma is caring for more than fifty grandchildren.

Some of the most vulnerable orphans are children of single mothers, especially if the mother is a prostitute. Because such orphans are from single-parent households, they may be neglected by other relatives. They refuse to provide any support to the children because they consider them illegitimate.

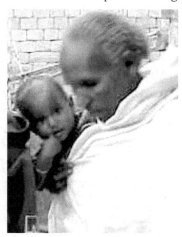

Pic. 2-2: Jember and his older siblings went to live with their Grandmother when his parents died.

Gelila, Mare and Dawit (Pic.2-3) left their one room zinc shack and went to live in town because of the constant abuse they received. Their mother was a prostitute.

Mare's mother, when sick, asked her to heat water on the open fire every night and to wash her feet with the heated water. She knew that her mother was very sick and needed her, but Mare's mother advised her to live with an aunt during her illness. She said that the aunt would take care of her. Mare feels guilty that she left her mother during her mother's last few days. She says that that this is the reason she misses her mother even more.

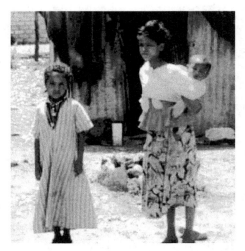

Pic. 2-3: Sick of being abused, Gelila, Mare and Dawit leave their zinc shack and take off for town.

According to her aunt, when Mare's mother was alive, she was able to provide everything, even basics like soap to bathe with. Currently there are days when not even soap is available to either bathe or wash their clothes.

Due to the decline of traditional extended family members, maternal rather than paternal relatives fostered Gelila, Mare and Dawit. When their mother died, the remaining extended family members avoided the children, which was extremely hurtful. They couldn't understand why their other aunts and uncles in the same village would not even look at them. The children put the blame on themselves. Gelila, Mare and Dawit desperately wanted to stay together as a family and not be separated from one another. Fortunately being able to stay with their aunt, they were in familiar surroundings, did not have to change their school, and could keep the same friends. Unfortunately, an important missing component to their life now is the absence of psychological counseling. Like the majority of AIDS orphans, they will never receive this crucial service.

Konjit, a woman infected by HIV, migrated back to her mother's home after her husband's death. She was in the later stages of her illness. By moving back to her childhood home, Konjit's hope was that her four children would find a male authority figure, such as a grandfather or uncle, who would give them social and emotional security. When she eventually died, her orphans were then twice disadvantaged. First they were traumatized by their parent's death, and then they had to adjust to unfamiliar relatives in a foreign place. But, this story gets even sadder.

The children were moved to yet another home to live with relatives and family friends where they all slept in the same hut. Tragically, the young girls were abused by the men. This happens in many instances and it is often the reason many women prefer not to accept orphan daughters from their own family.

Temesgen, Iskinder and Hassan (Pic. 2-5) lost both parents from the HIV Virus and had a difficult time being placed with relatives. Many children engage in migration when household members fall sick or die from AIDS. Little attention has been paid to the consequences that this constant migration has on their lives. Temesgen, Iskinder and Hassan were relocated four different times to live with family members. The boys were never consulted and often they would be taken to a new home many miles away during the night only to stay there for a few days. After a short time, they were taken to other relatives. Severed family ties exacerbated the difficulties faced by these orphaned children. Ultimately, they snuck out of the last location and traveled by foot for 5 km to the nearby town of Adigrat. When they arrived in the city, they had to live on the streets and were at extremely high risk of exploitation and HIV infection. Finally the Sisters found them sleeping on the street outside the gate of the mission and welcomed them in.

In nearly every sub-Saharan country, extended families have assumed responsibility for more than 90% of orphaned children. This traditional support system is under severe pressure, and in many instances has already been overwhelmed as it is increasingly impoverished and rendered unable to provide adequate care for children. UNICEF reports, most worryingly, that it is precisely those countries that will see the largest increase in orphans over the coming years.

What might be the best approach for those children who must migrate because their families have been affected by the death of their parents from AIDS? The children should be familiar with the place and people where they were moving. They should be included in family discussions regarding their migration preferences. And, there should be some way to maintain ties with relatives. This would ensure that children do not become distanced from their family and cultural heritage. There are currently a few organizations and programs trying to assist the orphans in these areas. One such organization is SOS Children's Villages.

SOS Children's Villages are committed to bringing up the children in its care to the best of its ability until they are young adults. They not only provide for the children's emotional stability, but also prepare them thoroughly for independence. Kindergartens, schools and vocational training are an essential part of the SOS Children's Villages. See www.sos-childrensvillages.org

"Rafiki" means friend in Swahili, and depicts the purpose of the **Rafiki Foundation**, i.e., to befriend orphans and widows in their distress (James 1:27). The mission of the Rafiki Foundation is to help Africans know God and raise their standard of living with excellence and integrity. Rafiki Training Villages provide educational facilities for orphans and vulnerable children in 10 of Africa's most impoverished nations. They also train African church partners in education, help them improve their schools, and support their widows. See www.rafikifoundation.org

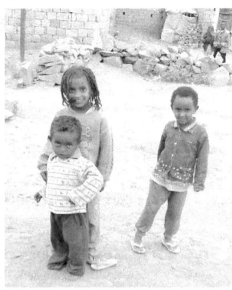

Pic. 2-4: Frew, Elene and Rada left their farm and came into town, Too young to be on their own, the Sisters have invited them to live at the convent.

Imagine you are nine years old, with three younger brothers and sisters, and you suddenly have no place to live and no source of income. Pic. 2-4 is the home of Frew, Elene and Rada. You are right: there is no home in this picture! They have been sleeping near that back rock wall. When her parents died, nine-year-old Elene became head of the household. The Sisters of St. Lucy have taken them into their hostel for the most neglected CHH. The children are together as a family and are given food, clothing, shelter and schooling.

The girls will enter a special program where they learn vocational skills that allow them to provide for their siblings. They actually pay the oldest girl to come to school, so she doesn't have to turn to prostitution to provide for her brothers and sisters. When the boys get older, they will enter the Salesian Vocational Center in town. The Sisters are trying to keep as many of these children together as a family unit as possible. You may wonder how these three orphans ended up homeless and sleeping in the street. Their story may seem all too familiar.

Frew, Elene and Rada left their home and farm on the morning their mother died, walking four hours down the mountain to look for help. When the Sisters of St. Lucy walked back up the mountain to make sure that the children's house was secure, an unscrupulous uncle met them to say that the property no longer belonged to the children because they had left. There were no deeds and the children had no legal recourse to get back what rightfully belonged to them. The three of them had no place to live, and by losing the farm, no source of income.

These children had always lived in a farmhouse, but they came into town when their parents died. Too young to be on their own, they've joined many others to live with the Sisters at the convent until they are able to go out on their own. As mentioned previously, there are organizations dedicated to mitigating these circumstances, such as the United Nations.

Many treaties endorse a policy that orphaned children should not be institutionalized, but should, where at all possible, grow up in some form of family environment. Growing up in communities disrupted by the epidemic, orphans more likely cope if they can live in surroundings that are familiar, stable and as nurturing as possible. Many believe that orphans should be cared for in family units through extended family networks, foster families and adoption. UNAIDS states that, at the very least, siblings should not be separated.

The UN proposes that adequate housing is a human right. Therefore, the pressure on international governments to provide adequate housing is gaining strength. Other issues inevitably arise where housing is poor. They include lack of food, access to clean water, forced eviction, gender discrimination, poor health, unemployment, low income or no income, and urban migration. Children are particularly vulnerable to the impacts of these issues.

Those older children fortunate enough to find some kind of work have to pay a high proportion of their income on rent, water, and electricity. This has a direct bearing on how much income is left over to meet the children's food requirements. You can rent a house for $3 a month. It is a 6x4 foot cement box only, no bathroom and no window. In many nations, in the rural parts of the country, the Catholic School is free, but you must pay tuition at the public school. So the Catholic Schools are full and they also provide breakfast to the children.

Many groups are starting to help the children. Habitat for Humanity International, in partnership with Nurturing Orphans of AIDS for Humanity, has secured a $600,000 grant from Comic Relief to build cluster homes for AIDS orphans in ten communities in Kwazulu-Natal, South Africa.

Most beneficial are the community and home-based care models that empower the affected children. They regard them as active members rather than just victims. Many children already function as heads of households and as caregivers. They are a vital part of the solution and should be supported in planning and carrying out efforts to lessen the impact of HIV/AIDS in their families and communities.

Despite concern about ethical dilemmas attached to the idea of children staying on their own without parents or adult supervision, it is possible with appropriate support systems for orphans to be nurtured in CHH. What makes it so difficult is that these children have no access to healthcare or education, and lack sufficient food, basic household goods, or agricultural necessities.

Time Magazine reported that by the end of the decade, it would take 80,000 orphanages that hold 500 children each just to house the children orphaned by AIDS in sub-Saharan Africa alone. This is what led to Robert Bland, Founder and Director of **Teen Missions International,** to start their project of bringing the "orphanage to the orphans." He described his method to me this way. They send graduates of their ten bible schools in Africa, into very remote areas. They build a small plywood building and are ready to go. They map out a five mile radius to their building and begin to help the orphans. They assist them in three basic areas: health, food and water, and education. Health-wise they provide basic first aid, malaria pills and whatever non-medical people can do for them. The malaria pills are so important. Did you know that three times more children die of malaria than AIDS?

Along with providing food, they also teach the children the basics of gardening and provide seeds and loan them tools so they can grow their own food. Clean water poses tremendous problems for the children. Some places have no water; some have just dirty water that the children have no way to purify. Teen Missions International has two drilling rigs in Malawi and Zambia that they bring to these remote areas and dig very deep wells so they will not go dry.

And for school, many of the children do not go to school because they cannot afford a uniform! Teen Missions International helps the children to get uniforms, pays their school fees and even teaches them how to sew, which then enables them to make more uniforms for others. Teen Missions International is a model organization that should be replicated throughout the world to help the CHH. Learn more at www.teenmissions.org and www.aidsorphans.org

Here is Temesgen (Pic. 2-5) He made a deathbed promise to his mom to take care of his younger siblings and keep them together. As a result of this promise, Temesgen, who might secretly want to see his siblings placed in foster homes, resists reasonable strategies suggested by relatives or child welfare authorities to do so.

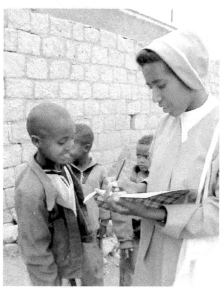

Pic. 2-5: Sister Desta helps a new CHH find food and lodging, and signs them up for school.

Like many other CHH orphans, the main reasons Temesgen and his siblings do not want to live with extended family members are:

- They do not want verbal abuse
- They do not want to be exploited for work
- They want to continue their schooling
- They feel that they are better off on their own
- Most relatives are very poor and unable to support them.

However, there are promising developments. Thousands of CHH are "rising." They live on their own, go to school, care for their siblings, and are on the way to a very good life. Many more can be put on this same great path if given the opportunity. It is up to the common person, you and me, to use our talents to help them.

3   What Do They Eat?

What would force Kidist (pictured below) to cook road kill for her siblings? Sadly, for children orphaned by AIDS, suffering hunger is a stark reality that they face on a daily basis. Poor nutrition contributes to more than a third of all deaths associated with infectious diseases among children under five years of age in developing countries. Good nutrition is essential. All children are happy when given food. Despite the sorrow of having lost their parents, these children continue on with a smile. Surely, at times the sadness overwhelms them, but normally they are out and about searching for food or whatever they need to survive for that day. Many survive off scraps of food they beg from strangers, road kill, or what they can salvage from garbage areas. Very young girls, 8 or 9 years old, often assume the heavy responsibilities of working in the garden, preparing and serving meals to both younger and older siblings in the households.

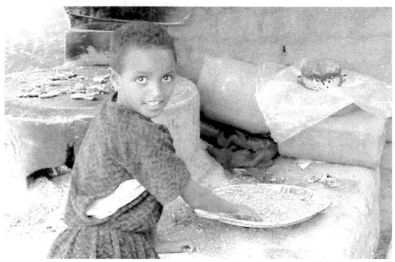

Pic. 3-1: Kidist provides road kill and corn for herself and her three younger siblings.

Kidist and her family live in their parents' farm home. The **Religious Teachers Filippini** give her a stipend to come to school, so she can provide for the family and continue her education. Girls who do not have this opportunity will often turn to prostitution to provide for the rest of their family.

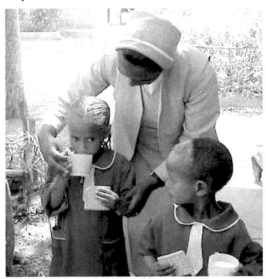

**Pic. 3-2: The first day of the milk program –
Samrawit and Bereket have never tasted milk before!**

HIV/AIDS-affected CHH without community support have very little food available for them. These children survive on so little. Most of them we have observed live on less than 1200 kcal per day.

At **St. Lucy School** in Adigrat, Ethiopia (Pic. 3-2), the children receive fortified biscuits and milk, and a hot lunch program when the funding is available. It is good to remember that it was the hot lunch program that ended grave hunger for children in the USA.

In South Africa, promotion of gardens is the most common food and nutrition service of programs for orphans. Twenty-seven programs have the children build their own gardens to grow their own food. These gardens aim to sustain the CHH and their families, as well as to generate income when excess harvest is sold. There is even one innovative garden program, implemented through **Africare** (www.africare.org), that encourages children to produce medicinal herbs in their gardens for personal use. Traditional healers assist in labeling plants in terms of their nutritional value, as well as their medicinal properties.

Orphans in Need (www.orphansinneed.org) has programs that distribute food parcels, which usually consist of tea, sugar, vegetables, spices, lentils, rice, flour and oil in countries such as Gaza (Palestine), Somalia, Senegal, Sierra Leone, Sri Lanka, Nepal, Kenya, Gambia, Mali, India, Kashmir, Pakistan, Bangladesh, and Afghanistan. Quite simply, they offer a lifeline.

More than 100 years ago Robert Hunter, with his 1904 book *Poverty,* tried to put light on the subject of childhood hunger and its effects on education in the US:

> The lack of learning among so many poor children is certainly due, to an important extent, to this cause (poverty). There must be very likely **sixty or seventy thousand children in New York City** alone who often arrive at school hungry and unfitted to do well the work required. It is utter folly, from the point of view of learning, to have a compulsory school law which compels children, in that weak physical and mental state which results from poverty, to drag themselves to school and to sit at their desks, day in and day out, for several years, learning little or nothing. If it is a matter of principle in democratic America that every child shall be given a certain amount of instruction, let us render it possible for them to receive it, as monarchial countries have done, by making full and adequate provision for the physical needs of the children who come from the homes of poverty.

The problem still exists in countless countries. Children orphaned by HIV/AIDS face a high risk of malnutrition and stunting. It is difficult to judge the extent to which orphans are becoming malnourished, because the sample sizes of orphans under five years of age are quite small. Research shows that the loss of either parent will worsen a child's height for age and increase their stunting. Researcher S. Kamanth published that there is accumulating evidence that early malnutrition, marked by stunting, is associated with long-term deficits in cognitive and academic performance, even when social and psychological differences are controlled. Stunting can lead to learning difficulties and poor health in adolescence and adulthood.

The United Nations Childrens Emergency Fund (UNCEF) analysis of 87 countries with recent available data shows that stunting rates among the poorest children are more than double those among the richest. All over the world, children living without permanent parental care are at a heightened risk of under-nutrition, putting their health and development in great jeopardy. Being homeless or surviving in inadequate and insecure housing has a direct bearing on someone's ability to feed himself. Children who are malnourished are smaller, more likely to get very sick from ordinary infections, and their brain development can suffer. Malnutrition is linked to nearly half of all childhood deaths. Government officials do not even have the means to determine how many children need help.

Food for Orphans mission is to supply at least one nutritious meal per day to as many orphans as possible. The estimate is that 400,000 orphans starve to death every year, yet with only 25¢, we can save an orphan's life. The type of food and nutritional support provided varies across programs from food parcels, to prepared meals, to food gardens or livestock donations. As they say, "Each meal you provide changes the future and offers hope!" (www.foodfororphans.org)

Peace Gospel serves orphans—they empower sustainable, locally-led, mercy-based programs in Asia and Africa. Their poultry project on the island of Cebu, Philippines has their hens laying a recent average of 1,134 eggs per week! The high demand for fresh eggs from local neighbors allows them to sell directly to the consumers on a daily basis. This makes their monthly net profit provide for so many orphans with food and education and also helps with some of the funding challenges of the organization. Learn more at www.peacegospel.org

When the Ebola outbreak ended, **Ambassador Ministries** discovered hundreds of children as young as two years of age living in landfills and city dumps throughout most of Sierra Leone. As they go into these areas. they bring as many children as they can to their Mercy Home orphanage to feed them and get them acclimated to normal childhood living. They provide financial and personal support for each rescued child in Sierra Leone. Learn more at amblp.ambministries.org

And where are the 153 million plus orphans going to get clean water? Over 4,500 children die daily from the terrible effects of drinking dirty water. Have you ever tried to live a day without water? Here in the US, we often take our water sources for granted, especially given we can drink clean water right out of our tap. In many countries, clean water is a scarcity and too expensive for the children to buy. Imagine trying to haul water in a bucket to your home each day if you have no running water. And you have walked miles getting water that is probably not even pure. Thousands of children fall ill daily from waterborne bacteria and parasites due to lack of clean drinking water.

Getting clean drinking water can be dangerous. Many children attempting to cross the road to buy drinking water get hit by cars. Most often, orphans can be seen drinking water from an old rusty, leaking pipe. Those pictured below are trying to get safe drinking water at a center set up by the **World Food Programme** (WFP), where large canvas bags filled with water are free to all who come and fill any container they have. The orphans' problem is that they have no containers. And the adults push them aside and block them from getting any water.

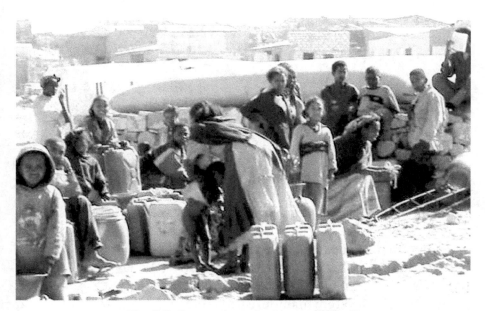

**Pic. 3-3: Access to water is very difficult
for the orphans because adults control it.**

All of the cash-strapped governments rely on international organizations like WFP to help feed their AIDS orphans. Many fall between the cracks and get no help at all. The food security of these children is a major concern. Lack of adequate land, know-how and water often drive the children from their deceased parents' homes to the cities in search of food.

Typical CHH families regularly go a whole day without eating, and are often hungry. Many are so anxious about getting enough to eat that they can't sleep nor do their school work. None of the CHH that we measure regularly eats a balanced diet. The risk is high that these children will never develop to their full physical and intellectual capacity.

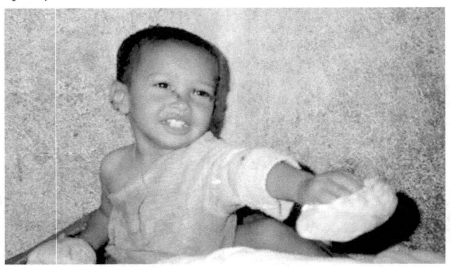

Pic. 3-4: Offering bread to his dying mother before he takes some himself.

Despite their own suffering, hungry children have a sense for those worse off than themselves. When I gave some bread to Ezra from Ethiopia (Pic. 3-4), he immediately turned to give it to his dying mother.

Many small groups and non-profit organizations are really making heroic attempts at keeping these children alive. Today, more children die of moderate malnutrition than from severe. In a sense, that is a great sign. The severely malnourished child is being helped. Our next challenge is to end all malnutrition. Many of you have heard the story of a young child walking along the beach picking up starfish and throwing them back in the ocean. An adult comes along and scoffs at him and says, "Why are you doing that? It makes no difference!" The young child replies, "It does to the ones I throw back." Natalie Simione, who runs Liberdade, where 35 AIDS orphans in Mozambique receive three nutritious meals a day, says it best for all of us caring for these children, "We can't save them all, but we will do our best with the ones we can reach."

Msizi Africa was established in 2007 after Lucy Caslon spent time with 50 orphans and vulnerable children at an orphanage in Lesotho,

South Africa. They have introduced more fruit, vegetables and meat to the children's daily diet, which brought health benefits and had a positive impact on their lives. Within a short space of time, they had more energy, were able to concentrate better at school and really benefit from their education. Now Msizi cares for over 1,000 children in Lesotho. Please see www.msiziafrica.org.uk

Several programs provide CHH the opportunity to own livestock, such as chickens or goats. These animals and their by-products (e.g., eggs and milk) are then used by the children either for consumption or sold to generate an income. A goat, cow, chicken or rabbit combined with the training received could benefit an orphan for the rest of his or her life. Such training gives the children the confidence and skills necessary to earn a living and have a secure future.

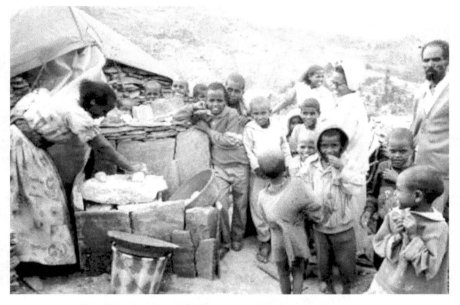

Pic. 3-5: Outdoor kitchens provide for all who come.

These children (Pic. 3-5) have arrived at an outdoor shelter where the Sisters provide a good hot meal for the children living alone out under the stars.

4   How Do They Survive?

"When our parents died, our relatives ran away from us. This surprised us because, being our relatives, we thought they would care for us. Our parents had a big farm, but it was taken from us so we had nowhere to grow food. My younger brothers and sisters became beggars. They would walk from house to house, asking for food."

Not uncommonly these days, and contrary to tradition, some relatives may take the property of the deceased parent and leave the family to fend for themselves. This situation could be avoided if people who are dying were persuaded to make a written will.

The need for money to purchase food and clothes usually leads the children to beg. They face a violent and uncertain life on the streets, where sex often buys food. Children will sometimes resort to prostitution and crime in order to survive. Grievously, rampant sexually transmitted diseases leave orphans at risk of becoming infected with HIV.

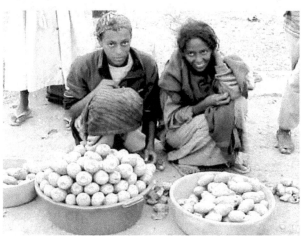

Pic. 4-1: Selling fruit is one way to survive

The growing phenomenon of Child-Headed Households scraping for survival shows the determination of the remnants of families to stay together, living off the kindness of strangers and the scant attention of social workers. This lack of full-time support forces them to engage in a variety of casual jobs to earn a living. Often exploited and taken advantage of, the children lose trust in the society that is supposed to protect them. The children, especially the eldest, grow up overnight to face adult responsibilities and the harsh realities of life. They must care for younger siblings, with hardly enough to survive on. And when they are adults, are they going to be willing to do this all over again as parents?

Vocational programs change lives not only for this generation, but for generations to come. The little boy in Pic. 4-2 was taught how to care for chickens by the Sisters when he was very young. Today he is thirteen-years-old and has a house and property with over 300 chickens. He is the "Mr. Tyson" of the area! He often returns to the school to provide eggs for the children. He also gives extra eggs so that other young boys can get started in the business.

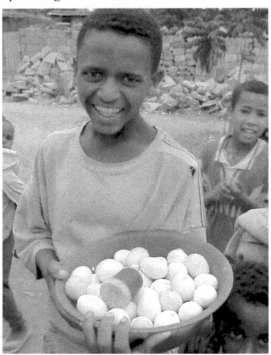

Pic. 4-2: Entrepreneur, since the age of 6, he provides for himself and three siblings.

Once enrolled in school, most of the children are able to complete their primary education. Sadly, because secondary education is more expensive, the older children are more likely to be forced to drop out before they graduate. As stated earlier in Chapter 2, in many places, the Catholic School is free, but you must pay for the public school. Unfortunately, while many NGOs and other groups offer support for primary education, this is unavailable for secondary school. The older siblings are glad that the younger children attend school because it frees them to go to work. The FOST Study found that secondary school fees are normally at least ten times the price of primary school. There's also much more pressure to wear a school uniform and purchase books and stationery in secondary school.

Several schools have programs that allow young children to complete their elementary school education while also learning a trade. In this picture (Pic. 4-3), Elisa and her friend show the Sisters their handwork that will be sold. Her earnings will help raise her three younger siblings. St. Lucy School will continue to educate her, and hundreds like her, until she is old enough to live on her own with her younger brothers and sisters.

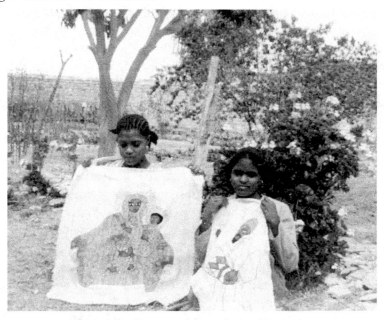

Pic. 4-3: Elisa and her friend with handwork.

Many of the orphan girls obtain an elementary school diploma, as well as a certificate in a skill that will help them earn a living in an honorable manner. They will be able to support not only themselves, but also provide for their younger siblings. The schools may help them set up their own micro-enterprise or find a good job in the city.

While some of the girls are not ready for higher education, many are hoping to continue on to secondary schools. The focus of The **Oprah Winfrey Leadership Academy** for Girls in South Africa has expanded its mission, and now helps the school's graduates acquire a higher education. This is a wonderful program. How I wish that she, and those with the financial means, could set up vocational programs for girls throughout Africa!

Uganda's Women's Effort to Save Orphans (UWESO) has been providing training and one hundred dollars in credit to female guardians of CHH to establish a small business. As of today, hundreds of thousands of orphans across many districts in Uganda have benefitted from this great work.

SOS Children's Villages is the largest charity for orphaned children worldwide: it operates over 500 villages in 133 countries, and has raised over 80,000 children. They help children with education, family strengthening, medical, and community outreach programs. They estimate that there are 153 million children worldwide, ranging from infants to teenagers, who have lost one or both parents. Learn more at sos-usa.org.

Martiny Family Missionaries has the Skills for Life Foundation (www.skillsforlifefoundation.net), which works to provide educational and vocational training to underprivileged and orphaned children in Guatemala. They provide practical life skills that enable orphans to achieve a better quality of life and acquire gainful employment. The Foundation fosters positive qualities such as self-confidence, motivation, and integrity to help children overcome the marginalization and resulting lack of self-esteem often prevalent in impoverished communities.

Their current programs include: Culinary arts classes, Pre-Engineering, and Carpentry & Woodworking. They even offer Micro-enterprise and Entrepreneurship. This is an important part of their vocational training programs, because as students produce, sell, and receive money from the products they make, they are simultaneously learning important business skills. Learn more at missionarytim.com.

Orphans need help, not only with formal schooling, but also with guidance on how to live decently. They must be taught the values that will carry them through a good and productive life. It's important to instruct them, at a very young age, how to seek help from nearby organizations, learn marketable skills, and how to run their own business. Many of you feel that you have nothing to offer these children, but you have a wealth of life knowledge that you can pass on to them. Volunteering for even a few weeks to teach these children, or to teach their teachers, could make all the difference in their lives. Simple marketing skills that we take for granted are so needed. The children are quick to learn and to implement all that you have to offer.

The kind of help the children need includes:

- Practical nutritional and health assistance
- Financial or material assistance and ensuring the security of tenure of the family in the house
- Developmental, emotional, spiritual and social support
- Ensuring that education, training and recreational needs are met
- Lobbying for free education for households below a certain income
- Facilitating guardianship arrangements
- Training in agriculture and tending animals.

Brittany's Hope is another organization dedicated to helping orphans. They recently established the HOPE Project (Helping Orphans by Providing Education), which gives funds to orphans, enabling them to attain higher education or trade skills. Visit their website, read about the project, and see how you might use your talents to help them. Learn more at brittanyshope.org

Sometimes, volunteers complain that the children seem ungrateful. It's not ingratitude. They've just never been taught how to express their gratitude. When you speak to them alone, they tell you of their deep feelings of gratitude to the many people who help. When I was putting a pair of socks on one child, she asked me how someone could be so kind as to send her these beautiful socks. Yet, she had never said a word when the socks were handed to her.

Many of the children have inherited the deep faith of their families, who have faced adversity generation after generation. They know they have to persevere, both for themselves and for their little siblings as well. And they will!

"The pain some children must endure in living their simple lives is beyond belief. Their courage can add meaning not only to their lives, but to ours as well if we have the eyes to see it, the ears to hear it and the heart to embrace it."

Wicks, Robert J., *Seeds of Sensitivity*

5 What's Best for Them?

"Over 13.4 million children are living without one or both parents due to AIDS."

January 2017 PEPFAR
(the President's Emergency Plan for AIDS Relief)

> Why? How are there still so many orphans?
> UNICEF tells us that every two minutes,
> an adolescent between the ages of 15 and 19
> is infected with HIV.
> Two-thirds of them are girls!

The Executive Director of UNICEF, Anthony Lake, pleads to the world:

> We need to finish the job of preventing mother-to-child transmission by providing lifelong HIV treatment to 95% percent of pregnant women living with HIV by 2018 and maintaining support for them throughout their lives. Fortunately, there is no mystery about what to do. This is a disease that we know how to prevent and treat, and new innovations are increasing our ability to reach children and communities living far from clinics and medical care. We are in a position to change the story—and finish the fight.

Mr. Lake's remarks reflect that same challenge proffered by the Joint United Nations Program on HIV/AIDS (UNAIDS), which states "The world is embarking on a Fast-Track strategy to end the AIDS epidemic by 2030. To reach this visionary goal after three decades of the most serious epidemic in living memory, countries will need to use the powerful tools available, hold one another accountable for results, and make sure that no one is left behind."

Will this strategy be enough to save the next generation of Sub-Saharan African children from becoming a nation of orphans? Today, right now, what is best for them?

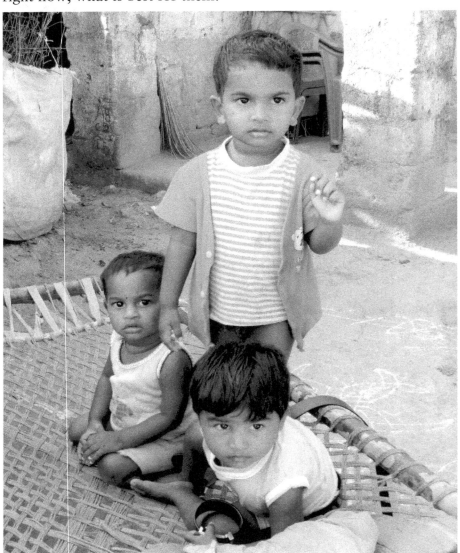

Pic. 5-1: What's best for them...?

Throughout Sub-Saharan Africa, there have always been traditional systems in place to take care of children who lose their parents for various reasons. Sadly, the onslaught of HIV has slowly eroded this good traditional practice. The spread of the disease undermines the caring capacity of families and communities. Deepening poverty due to lack of jobs and the high cost of medical treatment and funerals has greatly reduced the ability of friends and family to help these orphans.

Several things can happen to children when their parents die from HIV and AIDS-related causes. They may be absorbed and assimilated into another existing family, usually that of a female relative. Grandmothers and even great-grandmothers are taking on the responsibility of looking after the orphans of their deceased children. This is the ideal outcome, because it often means that there is minimum disruption in the children's lives after the death of their parents. But again, because of increasing widespread poverty and economic hardships, this is happening less and less. Eventually, the older generation will be unable to cope with the tremendously large number of children in need. This is why adoption or fostering of CHH is essential. **Children who are not with relatives must be a priority.**

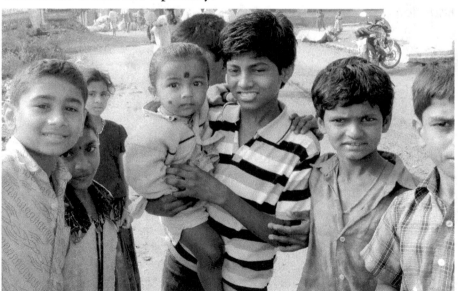

Pic, 5-2: No relatives to care for them.

When a dying parent can no longer care for them, children might be sent away from home prior to their parent's death. The ailing parents hope that their children will find better education and economic opportunities, as well as a caring home. Many families happily accept these orphaned children, because they become domestic servants. Girls are chosen in anticipation that they'll eventually get married and move away from the home. They don't become permanent members of the home, nor do they pose long-term competition for family resources with the caregiver's own children.

This deeply rooted tradition of child fostering within the extended family is one of the main reasons for the slow development of adoption in much of Africa. In some contexts, taboos and cultural beliefs may discourage people from taking children who are not relatives into their home. In Zimbabwe, the fear of invoking *ngozi* (the avenging spirit) is strong. In South Africa, obstacles such as tribal allegiances diminish adoptions.

On a more positive note, some anecdotal evidence suggests that fostering and adoption by unrelated families may have increased without any external support. This happened after the genocide in Rwanda where many families fostered unrelated children. The fostering was perceived to be a moral imperative, because so many children were orphaned.

If adoption within Africa continues to move slowly, what are the alternatives for taking care of these orphans? **America World Adoption** (https://awaa.org) reports that as of January 9, 2018, the Ethiopian government will ban international adoption from Ethiopia. This country has an estimated 4.3 million orphans. Institutional and residential care, such as orphanages and community-base projects, has proven to be successful, but both come with their own challenges.

Institutional and Residential Care

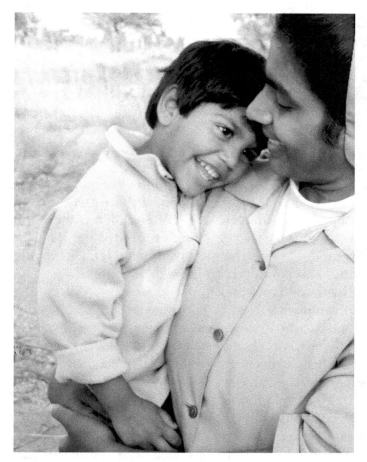

Pic. 5-3: Orphanages are sometimes the best solution.

"In dismantling the orphanage system, Progressive reformers laid the groundwork for modern welfare—the same welfare system that some reformers today want to fix (you guessed it!) by bringing back the orphanage."

Dale Keiger, Assoc. Ed., *Johns Hopkins Magazine*, 2017

Matthew Crenson's book, *Building the Invisible Orphanage: A Prehistory of the American Welfare System*, examines how the turn-of-the-century Progressive Movement championed childcare reforms that led to the dismantling of the orphanage system. He writes, "People are going to give me an argument about this, but I believe that in the process of dismantling the orphanages, what society did, albeit indirectly, was activate the institutional apparatus for welfare."

Orphanages, hospices, and other institutions in most developing countries have the estimated capacity to take perhaps five percent of all orphans into institutional care. In comparison, Africa's institutional care for orphans is quite limited. Only one to three percent of orphans are cared for in institutional settings. With the sharp increase in orphans in Africa, and the process of deinstitutionalization, new and innovative forms of institutional or semi-institutional care have emerged, such as children's homes and children's villages. They vary widely in size, management, and effectiveness.

Governments also try to offer support through programs such as adoption and fostering stipends, public welfare assistance, and access to education and health services for poor children and families. Even with these programs in place, countless needy families lack access to such government safety nets. Governments still generally rely on communities and volunteers to provide the bulk of social services for AIDS orphans and families.

The hardships faced by AIDS orphans have been documented for decades, and African governments are trying to develop and implement solutions. Some have created new laws and policies to protect children, and to also help women and children defend their inheritance and rights to property. They've also provided child advocates to help children redress exploitation.

Numerous books offer insight into the complex issue of orphanages. One is *Second Home: Orphan Asylums and Poor Families in America,* by Timothy A. Hacsi. His book is a well-researched and adeptly written account of the rise and decline of orphan asylums in America. It's a heartfelt and subtle argument about the best ways in which a society can care for its dependent children. As orphan asylums ceased to exist in the late twentieth century, interest in them dwindled as well. Yet, from the Civil War to the Great Depression, America's dependent children—children whose families were unable to care for them— received more aid from orphan asylums than from any other means. The asylums spread widely and endured because different groups— churches, ethnic communities, charitable organizations, fraternal societies, and local and state governments—could adapt them to their own purposes.

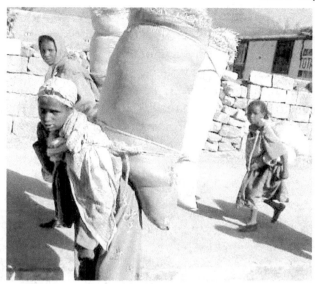

Pic. 5-4: Some kids work harder than others.

Another excellent book is Richard McKenzie's *Home Away from Home: The Forgotten History of Orphanages*. McKenzie, a business professor at the University of California, grew up in an orphanage in North Carolina. Upon polling hundreds of orphanage alumni, he found them to be happier, healthier and wealthier than the average American! His data supports the premise that orphanages and similar models, when run properly, provide an excellent solution to finding homes for displaced children in many parts of the world.

Africa can certainly benefit from well-run institutions, such as orphanages, to care for its displaced children and orphans. Malawi, Africa, is thought to have nearly 500,000 children who have lost one or both parents to HIV/AIDS. **Save the Children** in Malawi mobilizes and helps more than 200 village committees that care for about 23,000 orphans and others in AIDS-stricken areas. The program is serving as a model for similar efforts in Ethiopia, Mali, and Mozambique.

In Malawi, orphans placed in orphanages have an advantage over those placed in foster homes. These advantages include dimensions of lodging, health care, food quantity and variety, clothing and school supplies. Orphanage residents view their caregivers as compassionate and loving. Additionally, children in orphanages have more autonomy and a broader concept of their future potential. These institutions range from houses in the townships and suburbs looking after several children, to elaborate 'villages' with several houses, schools, playground and clinics. These are not the dark, evil institutes from the past, which you've often seen portrayed in the movies. Caring individuals, families, NGOs, churches, missions, and other charities run these charitable housing facilities.

It has been found that orphanages are more efficient in providing care and exchanging information with other organizations. Orphanages are also easier to replicate for use in other areas than are community-based programs.

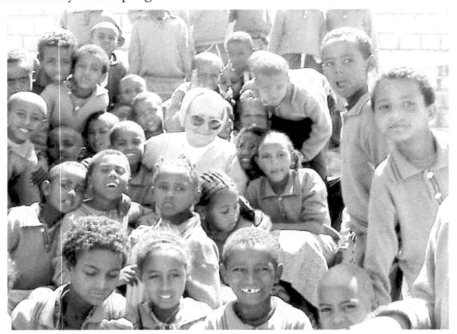

Pic. 5-5: Sr. Antonia enjoying the children she has been helping for 40 years.

In a somewhat ironic twist, the effectiveness of the traditional African social system in absorbing millions of vulnerable children has contributed to the complacency of governments and agencies in addressing the orphan crisis. Given the degree of national debt and poverty most African governments already face, many shy away from increasing the number of orphanages or other forms of institutional care. This is because it is economically impossible, and not because of the advantages of one over the other. For example, caring for a child in an Ethiopian orphanage costs $300 to $500 per year—more than three times the nation's average per capita income. Because of this economic issue, community-based support projects, rather than orphanages, are becoming common.

What's Best for Now?

This debate, fueled by the challenge of how to care for the rapidly increasing numbers of orphans due to the HIV/AIDS pandemic, largely focuses on two main models—"community based" care, and "residential or institutional" care for children. Despite data showing the advantages to children in institutional care, is it the expense that impedes the growth of orphanages? Or, are the community-based projects (rather than orphanages) really better for the upbringing of a child? Gill Grant, an advisor at World Vision, believes that the general consensus, noted from the extensive discussions on international internet forums, seems to favor strengthening community-based family care. However, some practitioners whole-heartedly advocate that there is a place for appropriate residential care for children. Grant advocates that it does not have to be exclusively one form of care or the other—there's a place for both.

A critical need is to develop sustainable community-based models that address the scale of this problem and provide quality and comprehensive care. Save the Children UK, and local governments, developed a program of Orphans and other Vulnerable Children (OVC) care in one poor municipality in South Africa. Within nine months, they were able to establish and train childcare forums (CCFs) in all of the municipality's 34 wards. The CCFs are community groups, whose role is to identify vulnerable children, mobilize community support for them, and link them to services and resources.

The chart in Pic 5-6 (see following page) compares global numbers of vulnerable children living with HIV to those in Eastern and South Africa.

	Global		East and South Africa		
	Female	Male	Female	Male	% of Global Total
Children living with HIV	880,000	920,000	520,000	540,000	59

Source: UNAIDS 2016 estimates.

Pic. 5-6: Children living with HIV (Global vs. Africa).

Janet Museveni, first lady of Uganda, has been assisting orphans for years in Ugandan resettlement camps where they are united with their extended families through OAFLA Uganda (Organization of African First Ladies Against AIDS). Museveni's organization also helps fund education and training for the children, in addition to providing credit to caretakers to start small businesses and trading activities.

There are now an ever-increasing number of orphanages, homes, transit homes and children's villages. These formal institutions that take in children orphaned by HIV should also offer programs to integrate them back into their communities at the earliest opportunity.

Let's continue to look at the pros and cons of institutional care more closely. One opinion is that institutional care is not a socially acceptable solution in the African culture. David Weiss, of the *Huffington Post*, blogged in 2016 that

> Three years ago, the government of Rwanda undertook the ambitious challenge of closing all orphanages within the country in an effort to provide Rwanda's orphans with homes with family members, or foster and adoptive families. In the last decade, with support from their national governments and donors like UNICEF and the United States Agency for International Development (USAID), additional countries have begun to implement deinstitutionalization policies.

Many African countries depend on a subsistence economy, and children sent from their village may lose rights to their parents' land. In addition, an institutionalized orphan is removed from the companionship of any remaining siblings and their community. In Zimbabwe, where AIDS has orphaned 7 percent of all children under the age of 15, the National Policy advocates that orphans be cared for by the community whenever possible and only placed in institutions as a last resort. Most surrounding eastern and southern African countries have also taken a stance against building more orphanages, because it drains resources needed to support family and community-based programs. Almost all Sub-Saharan African governments, international NGOs, development local policy makers, and practitioners have agreed to the description and position that residential care is "the last resort."

However, not only has there been no empirical basis for the above assertion, but, also, other care options have failed to make any significant improvements in the lives of AIDS orphans and other vulnerable children. In addition, we now know that formal placement of orphans with family members more often than not does fail; and, when it does, its impact on the orphan is devastating. The orphan completely loses trust in people and any organization.

Similarly, both non-statutory and formal residential homes have their problems. Traditional care systems are struggling to cope with chronic poverty, they can no longer be relied upon to efficiently and effectively take care of orphans and vulnerable children. In the end, we see that each care option has the potential to meet the needs, interests and rights of orphans and other vulnerable children. We must deal with each case on its own terms, taking into consideration contextual and structural factors that may promote or hinder care and service delivery to AIDS orphans and other vulnerable children.

6   What About International Adoption?

International adoption in the US is at its lowest level since 1982. The State Department reports that there were only 5,647 intercountry adoptions in 2015, compared to 22,726 in 2005. Even with this huge decrease, the United States still adopted more children through intercountry adoption than any other nation in the world.

Christianity Today reports that 80 percent of the drop in American adoptions can be traced back to three countries: China, Russia, and Guatemala.

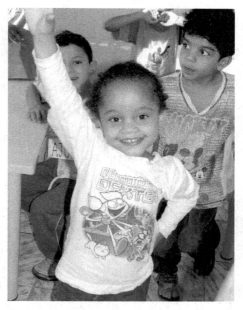

Pic. 6-1: The cutest ones get adopted.

China ratified the Hague Convention in 2006, which ensures that all international adoptions are carried out "in the best interests of the child." China imposed the following set of new regulations on foreign adoptions: banning adoptions by foreigners who were unmarried, over a certain age, over a certain weight, or taking antidepressants. *Priceonomics* quotes Harvard Law Professor, Elizabeth Bartholet saying, "The Chinese restrictions want to make a statement about how they're no longer a third world, but a first world nation. Insinuating, 'We can take care of our own kids. We don't need you.'"

The Russian government banned Americans[1] from adopting Russian children in 2012, leaving thousands of children in limbo and dropping the number of Russian adoptions from a high of 5,682 in 2004 to zero last year. The act to ban US citizens from adopting Russian children was in retaliation for the US Magnitsky Act, which punished a group of Russian officials who were implicated in the torture and death of a Russian lawyer named Sergei Magnitsky.

The decline in Guatemalan adoptions began in October 2007, after CNN correspondent, Harris Whitbeck, presented an investigation entitled *Guatemalan Adoption Controversy*[2]. Commenting on his findings, Harris said, "I was saddened for the Guatemalan mothers who either have had babies stolen, have been manipulated into selling or giving children up, or forced into doing so because of their dire socio-economic conditions. And, saddened too for the potential adoptive families who—only for wanting to bring a child into their lives and for their altruism—have in some cases become embroiled in sordid and shady dealings. There are no easy answers in this story and there are many, many layers to it. When I set out to report it, I did so to attempt to find the truth in what happened at Casa Quivira and the truth behind thousands of Guatemalan babies who have been exported to the United States."

Because of these many abuses, the Guatemalan adoption legislation was heavily reformed in late 2007 in order to be compliant with the Hague Convention. Subsequently, international adoptions effectively ceased in 2008.

Yet, there are still intercountry adoptions available. You just have to find the right group and have tremendous patience. Snow Wu, founder of Children of All Nations, has worked for more than a decade on behalf of China's abandoned children. Under Snow's leadership, Great Wall China Adoption has become a Hague-accredited international adoption agency that is nationally and internationally recognized for assisting the US and China in improving the adoption process and the laws that protect children. Because of her dedicated efforts for China's children, the US Congress awarded Snow the Angel in Adoption™ award.

---

[1] https://tinyurl.com/AIDS1000
[2] https://tinyurl.com/AIDS1001

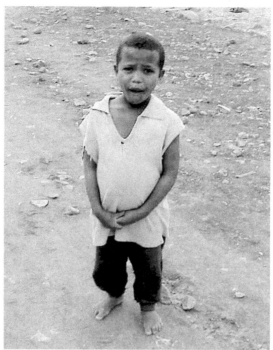

Pic. 6-2: If adopted, often children lose their language and culture.

Africa is another area where the US is still working on the international adoption process. There are also some misconceptions about adoption in Africa. Officials, at times, falsely claim that there are enough families within their own country to adopt or take care of the orphans. Although we wish this were true, when visiting packed orphanages, children's homes and other children's centers, we found that this is simply not the case.

Much of the resistance to international adoption is out of concern that children being adopted will lose their culture when placed outside their native country. But when a loving adoptive home is not available for an orphan within his or her own country, it's in the best interest of the child to be placed with any available loving adoptive home. It is important that families who adopt internationally, or transracially, actively take steps to teach their child about the culture in their country of birth. There is still such a great need for families willing to adopt these orphans.

Finding an International Adoption Agency

Having Hague Accreditation is paramount when searching for an international adoption agency. The Hague Accreditation and Approval Standards were created by the US Department of State. It is based on the provisions of the Hague Convention for Intercountry Adoption, the Intercountry Adoption Act of 2000, and the Universal Accreditation Act of 2013. The Standards are contained in the Federal Regulations that govern the Accreditation and Approval of Adoption Service Providers.

It will come as no surprise that not all adoption agencies are Hague accredited. There is constant policing to make certain that adoption service providers are acting in the best interest of both the orphan and the adopting family. An adoption agency can even lose Hague Accreditation. For example, the US Department of State temporarily debarred adoption service provider, European Adoption Consultants, Inc. (EAC) from accreditation on December16, 2016, for a period of three years. As a result of this temporary debarment, EAC's accreditation has been cancelled and it must immediately cease to provide all adoption services in connection with intercountry adoptions. It's critical that you perform extensive research on the group you're working with to adopt your child.

Proceed With Caution

Because they know that a picture is more likely to get parents to think with their hearts instead of their heads, unscrupulous agencies will often have photo listings of children. These agencies will take your money and provide you with nothing in return. Before you look at a photo listing, be certain that you are dealing with a reputable agency. Do your homework!

In addition to researching adoption agencies, there are a few basic steps to follow as you consider intercountry adoption. What age child would fit best in your family? Do you feel that you can accommodate an orphan with a disability, and, if so, what type of disability? Once you have made these important decisions, then and only then, look at your chosen agency's international adoption photo listings. The site, International Adoption Facts and Information[3], can help you make a good choice.

---

3 http://www.international-adoption-facts-and-information.com/

Exploring Sponsorship of an Orphan - AKA Adoption from a Distance

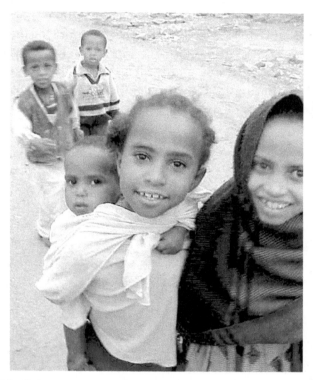

Pic. 6-3: Choose using information, not just the photo.

The great restrictions on international adoptions impel us to help children through such programs offered throughout the world. To participate in a program like this, a person sends money to a chosen organization each month. After that, they'll receive several reports and pictures each year from the child they have been supporting. The great advantage of this system is that the child is in his or her own environment and near brothers, sisters and any relatives who might still be living.

Angel Covers, like many other reputable organizations, uses the money you send wisely, providing food, medicine and education for the children. Angel Covers volunteers care for orphaned and destitute children around the world. Funds are raised through online product sales, generous donations, and grassroots fundraising efforts. They've been able to keep administrative costs at less than five percent, because they are completely volunteer run.

As discussed previously, it's wise to investigate the group you'll be helping. Inquire as to the percentage of your money that actually gets to the child. Sometimes it's better to give a monthly sum that can be designated for food, clothing, or education. In some parts of Ethiopia, the money you send for one child, even if only ten dollars, could buy bread for 400 children! Money goes a long way in these very poor countries, but, again, please investigate well.

7 Child-Headed Households Living by Themselves

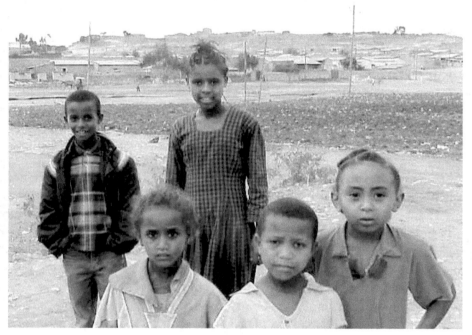

Pic. 7-1: Making it on their own.

We have been discussing placing AIDS orphans in some type of care, whether it is adoption, foster homes, or residential and institutional settings. But this book is meant to also focus on CHH who are out in the world making it on their own. They have a love of life and a deep love for their siblings. We need to give these CHH a chance to stay together as a family and make it on their own. An outrageous idea? Not if there could be adult supervision and a place where they can go for guidance when they need help. Supervisors can check them daily to make certain that they have all that they need.

There are too many successful Child-Headed Households to view them as helpless. What lies in the future for these AIDS orphans? We need to learn from successful children by examining their strategies to cope and move on to a great life. The silent power many children wield is that of resilience and endurance in coping with very challenging circumstances. It is possible, with appropriate support from NGOs and other community support systems, for orphans to be nurtured in CHH.

Again, it's important to remember that the advantage in the Child-Headed Household is that the children are not separated from their brothers and sisters to live with different relatives. Research in Zambia found separation of siblings to be a significant factor in psychosocial distress among orphans. Remaining in their parents' house is also a way for children to retain possession of their family's land, support themselves, and maintain a sense of continuity in their lives. In many cases, these children will continue to receive the support and guidance of the community.

Currently, 56 million orphaned children are living across sub-Saharan Africa. Only now has some empirical research begun to investigate the meaningfulness of life among this population. Few studies provide perspectives on the life-course consequences of losing a parent during childhood.

M.L. Goodman and his research team at the University of Texas Medical Branch at Galveston assessed life's meaningfulness in a cross-section of Kenyan women in early 2017. They assessed whether meaningfulness of life was lower among women who reported a parental death during their childhood. The study further assessed how this association was mediated by social support, family functioning, school completion and HIV+ status of household, and the extent to which lower subjective overall health among women who experienced orphanhood during childhood was mediated by less meaningfulness of life. They recommend further study on life meaningfulness and family capital in the context of the orphan crisis, and to promote equity across the lifespan. They encourage policy efforts to support orphans and vulnerable children. New policies should target strengthening support networks and family functioning to optimize self-reported health outcomes in determining how to best provide for these children. More studies such as these would be immensely beneficial to the orphan crisis.

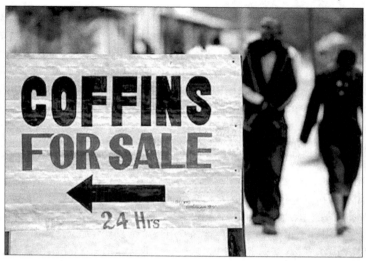

Pic. 7-2: One CHH business.

Many advocate keeping siblings together no matter what the circumstances. However advantageous, there are still times when it is not possible, or safe, for this. Becky Malecki, from Colorado State University, was once adamant about keeping displaced siblings together, but now offers some very strong reasons against this.

In the blog *Families by Design* Ms. Malecki writes:

> In the case of a relatively normal, well-functioning sibling group, they should be kept together—e.g., when a parent has died from AIDS or some other illness, and the children trust adults, then I would fully support it. However, in scenarios involving abuse and neglect, with resulting attachment disorder, I think keeping siblings together is often counterproductive to helping the children to heal.
>
> First, work on their healing. Keep them in contact with one another. When they are healed, then is the time to establish meaningful relationships. In other words, contrary to my initial beliefs, I now know that it's often absolutely necessary to sep-arate young siblings! Children need to bond to a loving adult in order to ever be able to deal with issues of trust, authority or real intimacy. A bond with an unhealthy sibling often stands in the way of the parent-child bond. It can be used as a crutch—*I don't need you, I've got my brother*, in much the same way gang members rely on each other for a sense of belonging and security.

The Religious Teachers Filippini, working with the CHH of Adigrat, Ethiopia, recognized that the very young CHH flourish best in a hostel or group home where they can still live together as a family, within the confines of a protected setting. These young CHH are provided an education while the older children are given technical skills so they will be able to make a living once they leave the Sisters. The Sisters do all they can to protect the children's inheritance, most especially any land that might be rightfully theirs. The children are encouraged and given the opportunity to visit any remaining relatives.

These children are assured of housing until they have a secure position in the work force, and are ready to be on their own. The Sisters have found that the older orphans, even though they have the technical skills, are not ready to be out in the world on their own all at once. The older girls are provided with housing within a compound. While living there, the girls can go to work, return to their own home, and live with other young women in similar circumstances. A Sister responsible for them makes sure that they have all they need. The orphans are counseled to help them transition to a life on their own as independent, caring adults.

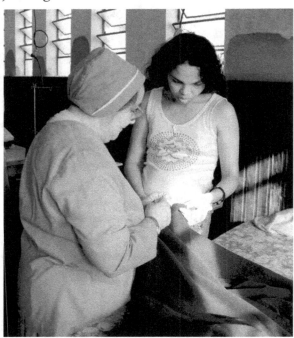

Pic. 7-3: Learning marketable skills.

As research indicates, it's inevitable that the number of CHH will increase tremendously over the next few years. With proper guidance, schooling and love, these children can grow to be caring adults with the ability to turn Africa into a productive continent. In order for these orphaned children to thrive and succeed, the world must remain focused on their rights as children and citizens. The African Charter on the Rights and Welfare of the Child (ACRWC) focuses on this need. From Article 25 of the African Charter:

> State parties shall ensure that a child who is parentless, or who is temporarily or permanently deprived of his or her family environment, or who in his or her best interest cannot be brought up or allowed to remain in that environment, shall be provided with alternative family care, which could include, among others, foster placement, or placement in suitable institutions for the care of children.

If this Charter had been adhered to, many children would have been able to thrive and to bring Africa to its proper place in the world. As of 2017, the ACRWC has been ratified by 41 of the 54 states of the African Union, and signed, but not ratified, by nine states. Four states have not signed the Charter.

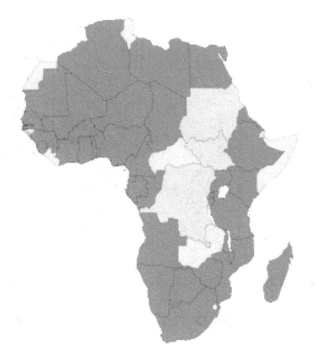

Signed and ratified: 41 states

Signed but not yet ratified: 9 states

Have not signed: 4 states

It is important to make children part of the solution in tackling the AIDS pandemic. Unfortunately, they are generally left out of the process when important decisions are being made. UNAIDS states that children and young people are virtually invisible in terms of public policy and of voices expressed on the national stage.

From Article 7 of the African Charter:

> Every child who is capable of communicating his or her own views shall be assured the rights to express his opinions freely in all matters and to disseminate his opinions subject to such restrictions as are prescribed by laws.

Ironically, children had no part in drafting the African Charter; nor are they being consulted on how to implement the articles.

Children's experiences of adversity are mediated by a host of internal and external factors that are inseparable from the social, political, and economic contexts in which they live. Serious doubt is being cast on the relevance of many traditional prescriptions for protecting children, especially interventions imposed from outside the child's social and cultural context.

The idea that children might take an active part in decision-making is still very novel. Some may fear the consequences. Frederick Luzze, former program officer with the World Vision in Uganda, is convinced that as long as the orphan crisis continues, and more and more Child-Headed Households emerge, the acceptance of the CHH as an alternative mode of orphan care is, for the time being, inevitable.

It is possible, with appropriate support from non-governmental organizations and other community support systems, for orphans to be nurtured in Child-Headed Households. The children need to be acknowledged as contributing citizens of the Africa of today. They cannot just be targets of interventions designed by adults far away from the everyday reality that confronts these children.

The UNICEF report, *Children on the Brink*, presents a simple strategic framework for action that emphasizes the importance of strengthening the capacity of children to meet their own needs as part of facilitating primary responses within a comprehensive HIV/ AIDS strategy.

Africa is only 13 countries away from making the ACRWC into reality. The health and economic problems of these African nations are overwhelming their capability to address the orphan issue. Those nations where most children enjoy basic good health, and are receiving an education, can help Africa in so many ways—if there is the will.

First Lady Janet Museveni of Uganda realizes the enormity of the orphan problem and urges all to sign the Charter. She says,

> The challenge of dealing with so many orphans requires dedication to ensure that what we articulate in terms of policy will provide quality interventions. Anything that affects our children affects our future. If it is bad, so will our future be. If it is good, so will our future be.

UNICEF estimates that there are between 143-210 million orphans worldwide. If there were a country comprised solely of orphans, it would be between 5th and 8th most populated country of the world. These numbers do not include unregistered abandonment as well as sold and/or trafficked children, but simply defines an orphan as a child who has lost one or both parents.

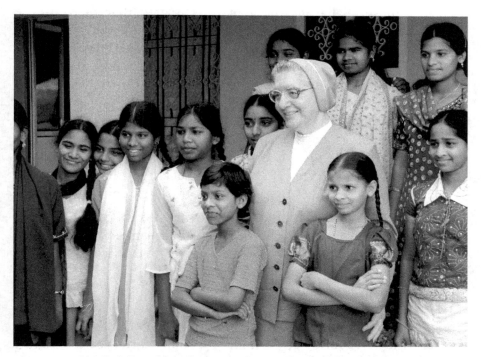

Pic. 7-4: Teaching them to take part in decision making.

Thankfully, along with the African Charter, there are several groups working for the rights of the children. The Rights of Orphans Project has as its mission to improve the lives of orphaned children worldwide by ensuring that each one can enjoy the rights guaranteed them by the Universal Declaration of Human Rights. This includes dignity, movement, social security, and property.

The SOS Children's Villages organization is also passionate about the recognition of children's rights: "Orphaned children all too often fall prey to abusive situations where they are sexually exploited, or they are forced to become child soldiers or child laborers. SOS Children's Villages' two-pronged approach of providing family-based care for orphaned children, as well as services to strengthen families, addresses these situations."

In an October 2016 speech, Dereje Wordofa, SOS Children's Villages International Director for Eastern and Southern Africa, highlighted the continuing plight of orphans in Africa when he said,

> In sub-Saharan Africa, it is estimated that there are 56 million street children and more than 52 million children who have lost one or both parents. Tragedies like HIV/AIDS, violent conflicts, abject poverty and natural disasters have taken a toll on families. That is why we need to work relentlessly to provide a loving home for every child who has lost parental care or is at risk of losing it. To succeed, we must be willing to work with communities, governments and international supporters to give children what they deserve: the chance to grow up with love, respect and security, and to strengthen the capacity of vulnerable families to care and protect their children.

For 60 years, SOS Children's Villages has been dedicated to the long-term care and prevention of orphaned and abandoned children. With 500 villages in 132 countries, SOS offers a family-based village model that provides for the holistic needs of a child—family, community, education and support—that are essential for a successful transition from childhood to adulthood. Through Villages, family strengthening programs, and other initiatives, SOS Children's Villages impacts the lives of over 1 million people each year. SOS are champions for the rights of children.

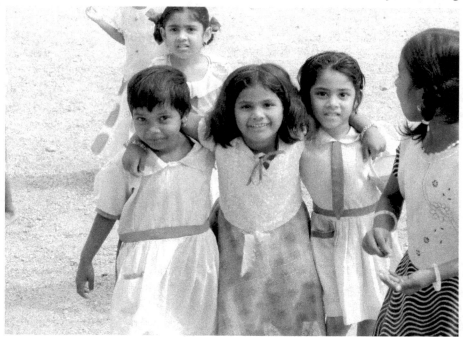

Pic. 7-5: Work for the rights of children.

Caution for the Rights of the Orphans

The world must remain vigilant for human rights violations against children everywhere. The Human Rights Watch Group reports one poignant example when, in 2016, the Senegalese government approved an initiative to remove children from the streets, including those forced to beg by their Quranic teachers. This initiative was an important step in reforming a deeply entrenched system of exploitation.

Human Rights Watch and the Platform for the Promotion and Protection of Human Rights (PPDH), is a coalition of 40 Senegalese children's rights organizations. The groups urged authorities to sustain the momentum with investigations and prosecutions of teachers and others who commit serious violations against children.

During the first half of 2016, at least five children living in residential Quranic schools died, allegedly as a result of beatings meted out by their teachers, known as *marabouts,* or in traffic accidents while being forced to beg. In 2015 and 2016, dozens of these children, known as *talibés,* have also been severely beaten, chained, sexually abused or violently attacked while begging. The deaths and other abuses highlight the urgency with which the government should penalize those responsible for abuse, and to regulate the traditional Quranic schools, known as *daaras*.

In June 2016, in a Twitter post, Senegalese President Macky Sall ordered that all street children should be removed, placed in transit centers, and returned to their parents. Anyone forcing them to beg would be fined or imprisoned, he warned. By mid-July, authorities had removed more than 300 children—including many *talibés* and runaway *talibés*—from the streets of Dakar. According to local activists and media, several other regions have also begun the initiative, which authorities plan to extend nationwide. Sadly, one year later, in May 2017 the group reported that the program has hardly made a dent in the alarming numbers of children subjected to daily exploitation, abuse and neglect.

More broadly, the program failed to trigger investigations or prosecutions of Quranic teachers implicated in forced begging and other abuses. Despite promises of sanctions by the president and the minister of Women, Family and Children, not a single Quranic teacher was arrested or prosecuted for forcing *talibé* children to beg during the first year of the program, which was carried out exclusively in the Dakar region.

The story does not tell how many of these children are orphans, and UNICEF has no data on its statistics tables for the numbers of HIV/AIDS orphans in Senegal. There must be thousands of them, and many of them living under these unfortunate circumstances. These orphans, the millions of orphan children of the world, who are living without any parenting, are the saddest human-rights victims of our generation.

Chapter 8 – What Will You Do?

> If I look at the masses,
> I will never act.
> If I look at the one, I will.
> **Mother Teresa**

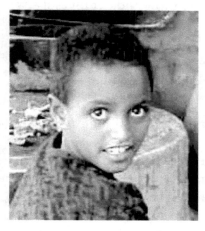

Pic. 8-1: What will you do?

If you've read this far, then you are serious in your quest to learn about children orphaned because of AIDS. That leaves me hopeful that you might also be serious about trying to help them.

Well, here is a young orphan you can help (Pic. 8-1)! She is the face of millions of children, not just orphans from Africa, but also from countries throughout the world.

The HIV epidemic shows no sign of disappearing. The world needs a strong wakeup call before the present orphans, and the millions more to come, grow up without not just the proper food, water, healthcare, clothes and basic education, but without love, a sense of belonging, acceptance or any core values. Most of all they need a "formation of the heart." There is not just one solitary solution to these problems. There are many solutions!

Governments are not the ones to solve this problem. While governments can provide the monetary and policy actions, the actual caring interventions for the children will need to be adapted to the culture and context for each child. This unprecedented crisis requires an extraordinary community response from non-government organizations (NGOs), religious groups and private initiatives. And, these groups must also be given the support they need to help the children.

In his Nobel Prize acceptance speech, former Secretary-General of the United Nations, Kofi Annan, said, "To live is to choose. But to choose well, these children must know who they are and what they stand for, where do they want to go in life, and why do they want to get there." The challenge is not to just avoid a catastrophe, but to ensure that these children be given the capability to make the best of their lives here on earth.

"If I give away all I have, and if I deliver my body to be burned but do not have love, I gain nothing." (I Corinthians 13) Not only will you gain nothing, but the children know when people are just throwing money at them. They need love more than all of your money. But how, you ask, can I give them love when they're thousands of miles away?

Pope Benedict XVI – *Deus Caritas Est*

Perhaps the words of Pope Benedict XVI, found in his encyclical, *Deus Caritas Est* (released 12/25/2005), will help you understand what you should do for these children.

> Practical activity will always be insufficient, unless it visibly expresses a love for man... My deep personal sharing in the needs and sufferings of others becomes a sharing of my very self with them... I must give to others not only something that is my own, but my very self. I must be present personally in my gift.

> We contribute to a better world only by personally doing good now, with full commitment, and wherever we have the opportunity. The Christian's program, like the program of the Good Samaritan, is "a heart which sees." The heart sees where love is needed and acts accordingly.

> Following the example given in the parable of the Good Samaritan, Christian charity is, first of all, the simple response to immediate needs and specific situations: feeding the hungry, clothing the naked, caring for and healing the sick, visiting those in prison, etc. There will never be a situation where the

charity of each individual Christian is unnecessary, because in addition to justice, man needs, and will always need, love.

These children need love more than anything else, and government programs do not provide love. Love can come only from those of us who care. Whoever wants to eliminate love is preparing to eliminate man as such. There will always be suffering that cries out for consolation and help. There will always be loneliness. There will always be situations of material need where help in the form of concrete love of neighbor is indispensable. The State that would provide everything, absorbing everything into itself, would ultimately become a mere bureaucracy incapable of guaranteeing the very thing which the suffering person—every person—needs: namely, loving personal concern. We do not need a State that regulates and controls everything, but a State which, in accordance with the principle of subsidiarity, generously acknowledges and supports initiatives arising from the different social forces and combines spontaneity with closeness to those in need.

This love does not simply offer people material help, but refreshment and care for their souls, something which often is even more necessary than material support. In the end, the claim that just social structures would make works of charity superfluous masks a materialist conception of man: the mistaken notion that man can live "by bread alone," a conviction that demeans man and ultimately disregards all that is specifically human.

Pope Francis calls the orphans "little stars that light up the night." He said to them at an Audience,

> You, too, are a treasure for all of us, the most precious treasure that we are called to guard. Forgive us those times when we adults have not cared for you, and when we did not give you the importance you deserve. I know that sometimes, at night, some of you feel sad, I know that you miss your father and mother who are not here, and I know too that sometimes you feel very hurt.

He goes on to say that the family is the foundation of co-existence and a remedy against social fragmentation. Children have a right to grow up in a family with a father and a mother who are capable of creating a suitable environment for the child's development and emotional maturity. Every child has a right to receive love from a mother and a father; both are necessary for a child's integral and harmonious development. Respecting a child's dignity means affirming his or her need and natural right to have a mother and a father.

I am reminded of the words of our beloved Saint Pope John Paul II, a great example to all of us as he not only prayed for these children, but provided for their material needs by setting up special agencies within the Vatican to help them.

> Children's faces should always be happy and trusting, but at times they are full of sadness and fear; how much have these children already seen and suffered in the course of their short lives. Let us give children a future of peace. This is the confident appeal which I make to men and women of good will, and I invite everyone to help children to grow up in an environment of authentic peace. This is their right, and it is our duty.

He also traveled to 104 nations to visit with them.

But What Can *I* Possibly Do for the Orphans?

As you reach the end of this book, are you wondering how you can possibly help to make a difference in the lives of these children.

Winning the lottery would provide a great start, but perhaps we should focus on a more introspective approach. What do you have to give? What talent did God give you to share with the children of the world? Most of us might respond, "Oh, I have nothing special to offer." However, this is simply not true.

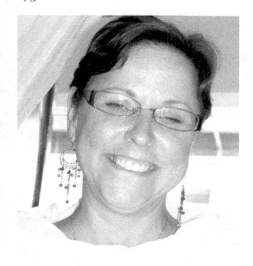

Pic. 8-2: "I can only play the flute."

Celine (Pic. 8-2) was quite like you. She sent me an email to say, "I would love to help the children, but the only thing I can do is play the flute." At the time, she was completing her doctorate in the flute! I wrote back saying, "Read your email—you can *only* play the flute!!" Celine used her talent and dedication to open a flute school as part of the St. Lucy School in Adigrat, Ethiopia, The children became so accomplished with the flute that they were featured on Ethiopian television.

Many were able to go on and support their siblings with their music. And, all of them received the joy of having music in their lives. When life is hard, if you have music and a song in your heart, you can face almost anything! Celine eventually became a professor at the University of Mekele in Ethiopia. And to think that the *only* thing she could do was "play the flute!"

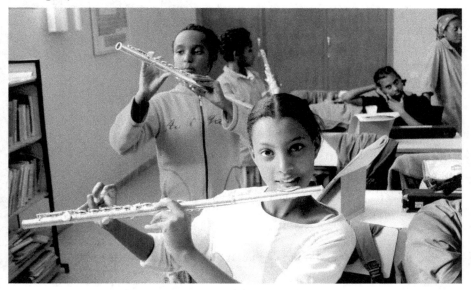

Pic. 8-3: St. Lucy Flute School Adigrat, Ethiopia.

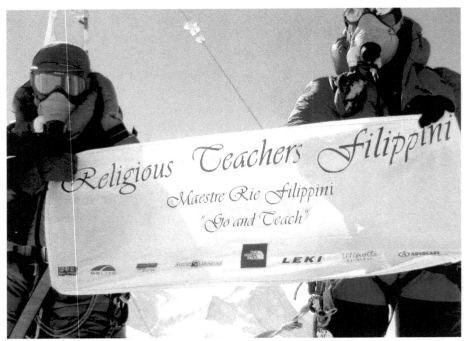

Pic. 8-4: Marshall planting the flag on Mt. Everest.

Marshall (Pic. 8-5) wrote and told me that he would love to help the children, but all he could do was climb mountains. Since that first email, Marshall has climbed Mt. Everest and the seven highest mountains in the world, placing the flag of the Religious Teachers Filippini atop each mountain.

Marshall had sponsors for each ascent who helped him raise enough funds to build an emergency clinic for the children in Hamelmalo, Eritrea. (Pic. 8-4) All that he could do was "climb mountains!"

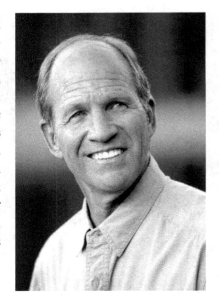

Pic. 8-5: Marshall – "I can only climb mountains."

And Lisa! (Pic. 8-6) All she could do was run! And how she has run for the orphans! She's run thousands of miles, raising money for food, clothing and schools throughout the world. Lisa was the first woman (Marshall the first male) to complete the ultra-marathon Badwater Quad.

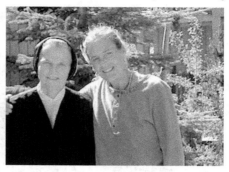

Pic. 8-6: Sister Mary Beth and Lisa.

The Badwater Ultramarathon[4] is a 135-mile course starting at 279 feet below sea level in California's Death Valley, and ending at an elevation of 8360 feet at Whitney Portal, which is the trailhead to Mount Whitney, Lisa has also run the Death Valley Quad, to the top of Mt. Whitney, four times. And if that were not enough to help the orphans, she ran 50 miles in every state of the United States in 62 days. And all she can do is "run!"

I'll end by telling you about a group of women in Charleston, South Carolina who love to sew. They, too, wanted to help the orphans, but wondered how to turn their desire and talent into action (see Pic. 8-7, next page). They began to sew dresses to be sent overseas. Now, thousands of dresses are sent to Ethiopia, Eritrea, India Brazil, Honduras, Guatemala, Haiti, Puerto Rico and Houston! (Pic. 8-8) Pretty impressive for a group of ladies who are all over 75 and only "know how to sew!"

So, what is it that you "can only do?" Take a moment to contemplate your talent or gift and please send me an email. The children need whatever talent God has given you. The orphans will benefit more than you will ever know and you will receive more than you might ever have expected.

> If I look at the masses, I will never act. If I look at the one, I will.
>
> Mother Teresa

---

4 https://en.wikipedia.org/wiki/Ultramarathon

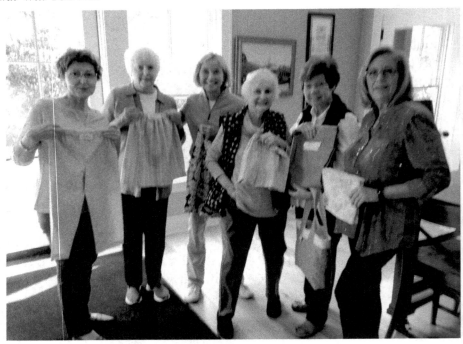

Pic. 8-7: "The only thing that I can do is sew."

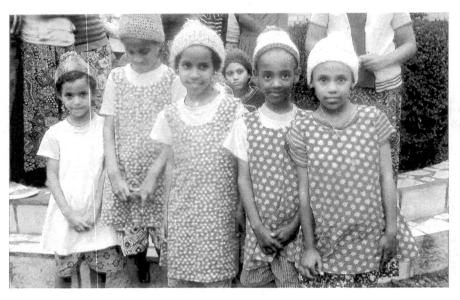

Pic. 8-8: Orphans model the dresses made by volunteers.

How Donations Make a Difference

Please know that 100% of your gift goes directly to assisting Child-Headed Households. The Religious Teachers Filippini would be glad to speak with you as you decide how to best help these deserving orphans. You are also afforded the opportunity to visit and stay with the children so that you may see how they are succeeding.

Child-Headed Households where the oldest member is over 12 years-of-age are provided small homes and then enter a program where they learn a trade. This enables them to earn some money right away for their family, while also studying for their elementary education diploma. They learn sewing, knitting, embroidering, gardening and how to raise poultry. They're also taught basic business skills to help their micro-enterprise be successful. The Religious Teachers Filippini will soon be opening a similar initiative for orphans in Addis Ababa.

For all donations, please make checks payable to Religious Teachers Filippini and mail to:

> **Sr. Mary Elizabeth Lloyd, MPF**
> **Villa Walsh Convent**
> **455 Western Avenue**
> **Morristown, NJ 07960**

Religious Teachers Filippini can be reached at (973) 538-2886

* The Religious Teachers Filippini is a non-profit 501(c)(3), tax-deductible organization.

Thank you

Prayer for the Child-Headed Households

Mary Immaculate Virgin, Woman of pain and hope, be benevolent to the children who suffer and obtain for them fullness of life. Turn your maternal gaze especially to those children who are in extreme need. Look kindly and help the grandparents who are without sufficient resources to support their grandchildren who have become orphans. Look at the siblings living together huddled alone never to feel a mother's touch. Clasp all of them to your maternal heart, and let them feel a mother's love. Most Holy Virgin, pray for us.

Appendix A: HIV/AIDS -- The Basics

Key Points

HIV is the virus that causes HIV infection. AIDS is the most advanced stage of HIV infection[5.]

- HIV is spread through contact with the blood, semen, pre-seminal fluid, rectal fluids, vaginal fluids, or breast milk of a person with HIV. In the United States, HIV is spread mainly by having anal or vaginal sex or sharing drug injection equipment with a person who has HIV.

- Antiretroviral therapy (ART) is the use of HIV medicines to treat HIV infection. People on ART take a combination of HIV medicines (called an HIV regimen) every day.

- ART can't cure HIV infection, but it can help people with HIV live longer, healthier lives. HIV medicines can also reduce the risk of transmission of HIV.

What is HIV/AIDS?

HIV stands for human immunodeficiency virus, which is the virus that causes HIV infection. The abbreviation "HIV" can refer to the virus or to HIV infection.

AIDS stands for acquired immunodeficiency syndrome. AIDS is the most advanced stage of HIV infection.

HIV attacks and destroys the infection-fighting CD4 cells of the immune system. The loss of CD4 cells makes it difficult for the body to fight infections and certain cancers. Without treatment, HIV can gradually destroy the immune system and advance to AIDS.

---

5 This appendix is taken from https://aidsinfo.nih.gov/understanding-hiv-aids/fact-sheets/19/45/hiv-aids--the-basics

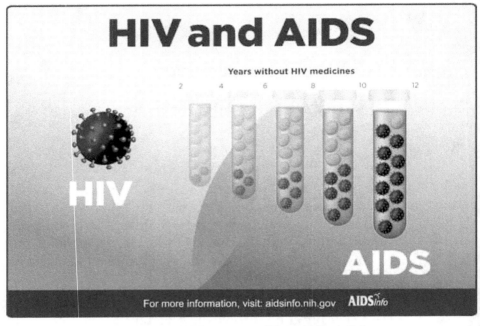

Pic. A-1: HIV and AIDS – Years without HIV medicines.

How is HIV spread?

HIV is spread through contact with certain body fluids from a person with HIV. These body fluids include:

- Blood
- Semen
- Pre-seminal fluid
- Vaginal fluids
- Rectal fluids
- Breast milk

The spread of HIV from person to person is called HIV transmission. The spread of HIV from a woman with HIV to her child during pregnancy, childbirth, or breastfeeding is called mother-to-child transmission of HIV.

In the United States, HIV is spread mainly by having sex with or sharing drug injection equipment with someone who has HIV. To reduce your risk of HIV infection, use condoms correctly and consistently during sex, limit your number of sexual partners, and never share drug injection equipment.

Mother-to-child transmission is the most common way that children become infected with HIV. HIV medicines, given to women with HIV during pregnancy and childbirth and to their babies after birth, reduce the risk of mother-to-child transmission of HIV.

You can't get HIV by shaking hands or hugging a person who has HIV. You also can't get HIV from contact with objects such as dishes, toilet seats, or doorknobs used by a person with HIV. HIV does not spread through the air or through mosquito, tick, or other insect bites.

What is the treatment for HIV?

Antiretroviral therapy (ART) is the use of HIV medicines to treat HIV infection. People on ART take a combination of HIV medicines (called an HIV regimen) every day. (HIV medicines are often called antiretrovirals or ARVs.)

ART prevents HIV from multiplying and reduces the amount of HIV in the body. Having less HIV in the body protects the immune system and prevents HIV infection from advancing to AIDS.

ART can't cure HIV, but it can help people with HIV live longer, healthier lives. ART also reduces the risk of HIV transmission.

What are the symptoms of HIV/AIDS?

Within 2 to 4 weeks after a person becomes infected with HIV, they may have flu-like symptoms, such as fever, chills, or rash. The symptoms may last for a few weeks after they become infected.

After this earliest stage of HIV infection, HIV continues to multiply but at very low levels. More severe symptoms of HIV infection, such as signs of opportunistic infections, generally don't appear for many years. (Opportunistic infections are infections and infection-related cancers that occur more frequently or are more severe in people with weakened immune systems than in people with healthy immune systems.)

Without treatment with HIV medicines, HIV infection usually advances to AIDS in 10 years or longer, though it may take less time for some people.

HIV transmission is possible at any stage of HIV infection—even if a person with HIV has no symptoms of HIV.

How is AIDS diagnosed?

The following criteria are used to determine if a person with HIV has AIDS:

- The person's immune system is severely damaged, as indicated by a CD4 count of less than 200 cells/mm³. A CD4 count measures the number of CD4 cells in a sample of blood. The CD4 count of a healthy person ranges from 500 to 1,600 cells/mm³.

AND/OR

- The person has developed certain opportunistic infections.

Where can I learn more about HIV/AIDS?

- **How Is HIV Transmitted?** from HIV.gov
  https://www.hiv.gov/hiv-basics/overview/about-hiv-and-aids/how-is-hiv-transmitted

- **HIV 101** from the Centers for Disease Control and Prevention (CDC)
  http://www.cdc.gov/hiv/pdf/library/factsheets/hiv101-consumer-info.pdf
  http://www.cdc.gov/hiv/pdf/library/factsheets/hiv101-consumer-info.pdf

This fact sheet is based on information from the following sources:

- From CDC: **HIV Basics**
  (http://www.cdc.gov/hiv/basics/index.html)

- From the National Institute of Allergy and Infectious Diseases (NIAID): **HIV/AIDS**
  https://www.niaid.nih.gov/diseases-conditions/hivaids

Appendix B: Orphans Mentioned in This Book: Traditional Ethiopian Names and Their Meanings

Ethiopian Name	English Meaning
Abeba	Flower
Becca	Understanding God
Bereket	Blessings
Biftu	Early Morning
Dawit	Beloved
Desta	Joyful
Elene	Light
Emebet	Respected First Lady
Feker	Love
Fisha	Joy
Frew	Seed
Gelila	Tempting Beauty
Jember	Sunset
Kidist	Blessed
Mare	Honey
Mekonnen	Honorable
Mimi	Desired
Rada	Our Helper
Samrawit	Unity
Temesgen	Thank Our Lord
Tsefy	My Hope

Acknowledgements

This work could not have been completed without the support and generosity of the following people. With gratitude and prayers I thank...

Sr. Nicolina Bandiera, MPF, Superior General of the Religious Teachers Filippini

Sr. Mary De Bacco, MPF, Superior General Emeritus of the Religious Teachers Filippini

Sr. Ascenza Tizzano, MPF, Provincial Superior Religious Teachers Filippini USA

The Teachers Filippini of Ethiopia, Eritrea, India, Brazil and Albania, Italy, and the USA

...and in alphabetical order...

Lisa Smith-Batchen

Anita Branch

Angelo D'Amelio

Noel and Virginia George

Heather Humienny

Gregory and Kathy Johnson

Lisa Lanterman

William Lloyd, MD

Mary O'Hara, MD

Maureen Lloyd

Sr. Margherita Marchione, M.P.F.

David McIntee

Margaret Meys

Rachel Barcia Morse

Lianne Latkany Russo

Andrea Schaeffer

Joe Vitale

Victor R. Volkman, CEO, Loving Healing Press

Jillian Coleman Wheeler

Christine Burrows Yi, MD

.

About the Author

"Everyone can help the starving mothers and children of the world – even if you only help a little!"

Sister Mary Elizabeth Lloyd, MPF, entered the Institute of the Religious Teachers Filippini when she was 18 years old. She taught science and coached interscholastic sports teams before continuing graduate school at Columbia University. After receiving her doctorate in Nutrition and Public Health, Sr. Mary Beth served at Memorial Sloane Kettering Cancer Center in New York City. It was at this point when the various pieces of her vocation as educator and scientist collided in a most providential way.

In 1994, Sr. Mary Beth responded to the Institute's need for an International Mission Office Director, a position she still holds today. Her ministry includes working with and helping to provide for the women and children served by the Filippini Missions in Albania, Ethiopia, Eritrea, India and Brazil.

Sr. Mary Beth's development activities transcend traditional fundraising. A lifelong athlete herself, Sr. Mary Beth has participated in numerous sponsored road races, marathons, and ultra-marathons to raise funds for the missions. In 2010 she completed consecutive 50-mile runs in all 50 states, a feat which generated global awareness of the Filippini ministry and the inspirational human-interest story about "The Running Nun."

In every city and village she visits, Sr. Mary Beth carries with her God's message of hope and the call for everyone to perform "one little act" to improve the world. Her passion for serving others struck a chord, fueled by extensive news media coverage including ABC's *Good Morning America*, CNN, and ESPN.

In recognition of her lifelong service to the world's neediest, Sr. Mary Beth was bestowed the title *Servitor Pacis*, "Servant of Peace," by the Path to Peace Foundation in a public ceremony held at the United Nations.

Sr. Mary Beth currently serves the USA Filippini Community Leadership Team as Councilor and Secretary in Morristown, New Jersey.

After reading this book you will never again challenge the notion *"What can one person do to make a difference?"*

This book has been written with the intention to inform as many people as possible about the situation of the AIDS orphans and their Child-Headed Households. I have made a great effort to recognize everyone whose works have been used to help explain this cause. Should you feel I have slighted you or any group please write to me, and I will make the proper insertions. **srmelloyd@gmail.com**

About the Religious Teachers Filippini

The Religious Teachers Filippini have been helping the poorest women and children survive for more than 300 years. In the recent past, our schools and initiatives for orphans and widows were developed mainly due to the consequences of war. Now the times are changing and we are adapting by providing these same survival and life skills to the Child-Headed Households. Many of our graduates in Ethiopia have gone on to set up their own restaurants or sewing shops. Others have become successful in business and technology or in teaching and nursing.

It is very touching to see the former graduates return with their own families to thank the Sisters for all that the Sisters have done for them. One memorable event was when one of our former students returned with dozens of eggs for the Sisters to feed the orphans. The former student recounted how he and his brother were starving when the Sisters took them in, and not only fed them, but loved, educated and provided for their every need.

For more information about the Religious Teachers Filippini's work, please visit **www.filippiniusa.org**.

100% of all profits from this book will go
to help the Child-Headed Households.

Donations to help may be sent c/o
Religious Teachers Filippini Mission Fund
455 Western Ave.
Morristown, NJ 07960

And they are tax deductible!

Index

CPSIA information can be obtained
at www.ICGtesting.com
Printed in the USA
BVHW091939011118
531828BV00001B/2/P

9 781615 994014